new keto:
dinner in
30

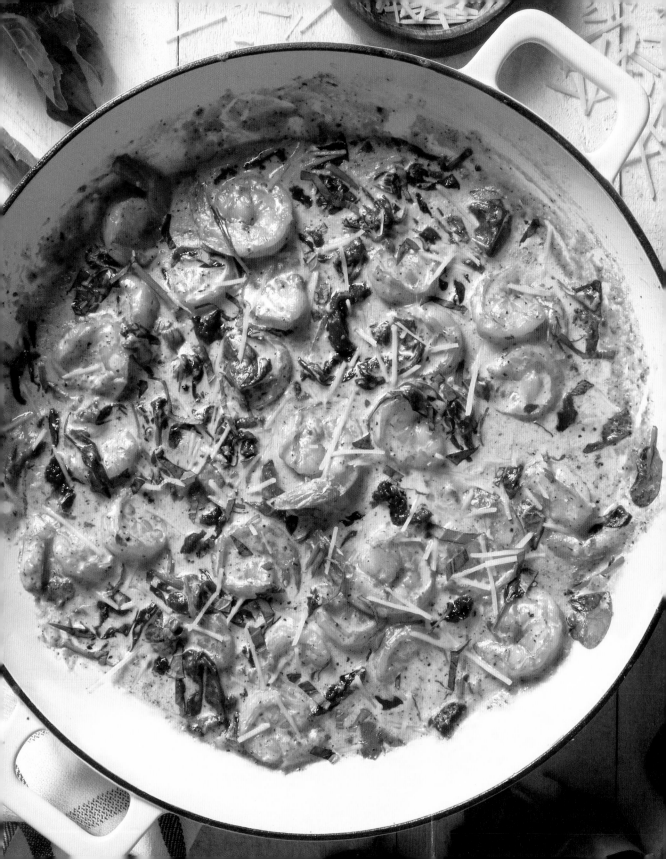

new keto: dinner in 30

Super Easy and Affordable Recipes for a Healthier Lifestyle

michael silverstein

Celebrity chef and author of *New Keto Cooking* and *New Comfort Cooking*

PAGE STREET
PUBLISHING CO.

PAGE STREET
PUBLISHING CO.

Copyright © 2022 Michael Silverstein

First published in 2022 by
Page Street Publishing Co.
27 Congress Street, Suite 1511
Salem, MA 01970
www.pagestreetpublishing.com

Distributed by Macmillan, sales in Canada by The Canadian Manda Group.

26   25   24   23   22   1   2   3   4   5

ISBN-13: 978-1-64567-900-4
ISBN-10: 1-64567-900-4

Library of Congress Control Number: 2022935240

Cover and book design by Meg Baskis for Page Street Publishing Co.
Photography by Michael Silverstein
Portrait photography by Dan Galvan

Printed and bound in the United States of America

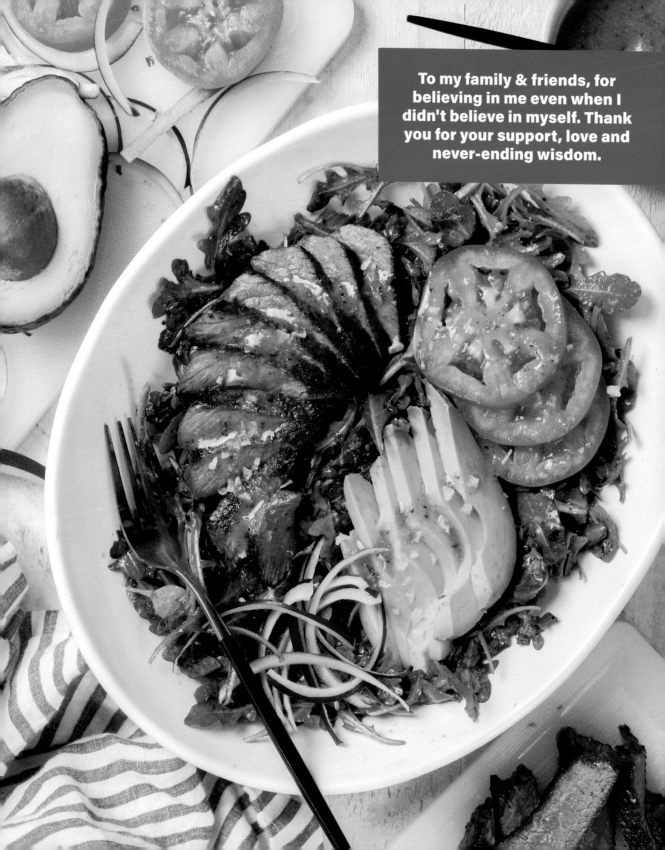

To my family & friends, for believing in me even when I didn't believe in myself. Thank you for your support, love and never-ending wisdom.

contents

Introduction 8

Deciding What's for Dinner 11

brisk beef 12

Texas Chili-Rubbed Ribeye
with Fiery Chipotle Butter 14

Bacon Cheeseburger Skillet
with "Big Mike" Sauce 17

Mouthwatering Mongolian Beef 18

15-Minute Heavenly Steak Bites 21

No-Frilly Weeknight Chili 22

Thousand Island Reuben Skillet 25

Finger-Lickin' Low-Carb Steak Tacos
with Smoky Crema 26

Mellow Mushroom Smothered Tri-Tips 29

Keto Korean Barbecue Short Ribs
(L.A. Galbi) 30

Blue Cheese Lovers' Steak and
Asparagus Sauté 33

Mediterranean-Spiced Kebabs
with Dill Yogurt Drizzle 34

choice chicken 36

Mike's Famous Bourbon Chicken 38

Firecracker Chicken Meatballs 41

The Perfect Garlic Parmesan Wings 42

Piece-of-Cake Chicken Bake 45

Zesty "Honey Mustard" Chicken 46

Low-Carb Barbecue Chicken
Tortilla Pizzas 49

Quick Chicken Parm 50

Thai Green Curry in a Hurry 53

My Big Fat Greek Sheet-Pan Chicken 54

Parmesan-Crusted Chicken Piccata 57

Chili-Lime Grilled Chicken
with Garlicky Aioli 58

pronto pork 60

Popcorn Pork Belly with Yum Yum Sauce 62

Austin Food Truck Breakfast Tacos (for Dinner!) 65

Spicy Italian Stuffed Banana Peppers 66

Amazing Keto Pork Fried Rice 69

Last-Minute Low-Carb "Al Pastor" Bowls 70

Vibrant Thai-Style Pork Larb 73

Pork Chops in Wicked Mardi Gras Sauce 74

suddenly seafood 76

Creamy Sun-Dried Tomato Tuscan Shrimp 78

Summery Grilled Swordfish
with Avocado Salsa 81

Date Night Spicy Tuna Sushi Boats 82

Kickin' Cajun Shrimp and Sausage Bake ... 85

Extra-Crispy Salmon and Green Beans with "Horsey" Sauce ... 86

Luxurious Low-Carb Tuna Pasta with Olive Oil and Lemon ... 89

Succulent Spanish Garlic Shrimp (Gambas al Ajillo) ... 90

Lemon Dill Salmon en Papillote ... 93

speedy soups & salads ... 94

Southwest Roasted Tomato Bisque ... 96

Easy Egg Drop Soup ... 99

Hearty Stuffed Pepper Soup ... 100

Comforting Keto Cream of Mushroom Soup ... 103

Simply Delish Sausage and Kale Soup ... 104

The Ultimate Blackened Chicken Caesar Salad ... 107

Steak and Avocado Salad with Sweet Onion Dressing ... 108

Loaded Lemon-Pepper Broccoli Salad ... 111

Protein-Packed Maryland Shrimp Salad ... 112

Blissful Burrata and Pancetta Salad with Summer Citronette ... 115

standout sides ... 116

Cheesy Baked Asparagus ... 118

Sweet Balsamic-Glazed Brussels ... 121

Blistered Sichuan-Style Green Beans ... 122

Fab 5-Minute Spanish Rice ... 125

Herby Pan-Roasted Mushrooms ... 126

Beautifully Layered Eggplant Caprese ... 129

Lemony Spice-Roasted Mixed Veggies ... 130

Fabulous Bacon-Fried Cabbage Steaks ... 133

swift sweets ... 134

Boozy Margarita Mug Cake ... 136

Seductive Strawberry Mojito Fool ... 139

Blueberry Lemon Mini Muffins ... 140

Chewy Ginger Almond Butter Cookies ... 143

Mike's Midnight Munchie Bars ... 144

chef's cheat sheet ... 146

Tips and Tricks: Saving Time and Money ... 148

Pantry Principles ... 150

Meat Matters ... 155

Knife Life ... 158

Acknowledgments ... 160

About the Author ... 161

Index ... 162

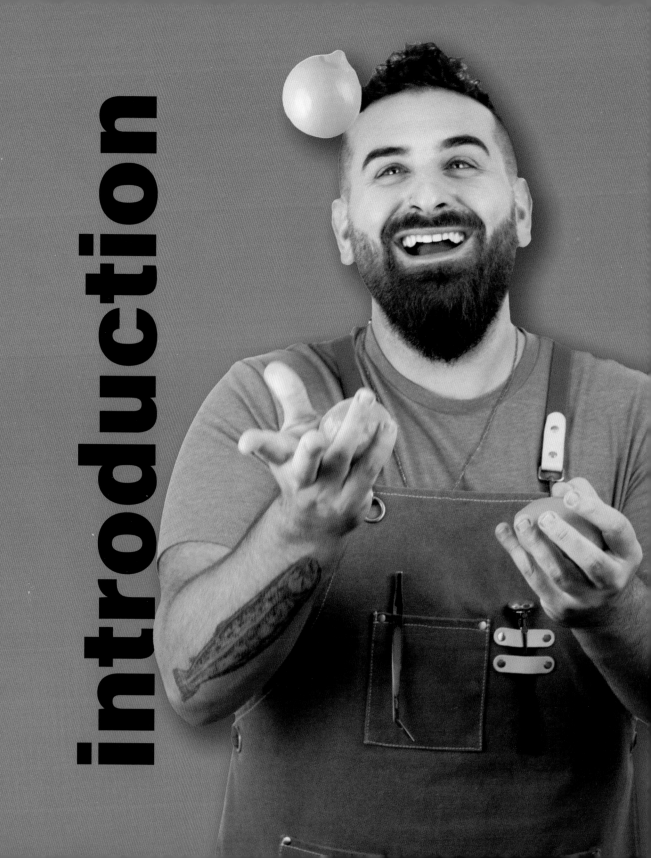

introduction

I have three words for you: quick, healthy and freakin' delicious. (Okay, fine. That's four words. But it's just how I feel . . .)

Look, it's time we moved past the idea that eating healthy means eating expensive, boring food. I'm tired of the common expectation that eating better requires sacrificing everything you love for your health. Most importantly, I'm tired of the idea that you need hours and hours in the kitchen every day to make beautiful meals at home. It's just not true, and this book is here to prove it. There is a way to make all your favorite foods—all the yummiest, most indulgent meals for you and your family—without sacrifice. And you can do it quickly and easily too. With this book, you'll be making restaurant-quality, Keto-friendly dinners in no time at all.

Even for me, after a long work day, I just need to get dinner on the table. And that food still needs to be 100-percent delicious. It also needs to be healthy and exciting. There are dinners in this book that you can make in 15 minutes. There are family-sized meals in this book that cost less than $10 USD. And all of them are low-carb, high-flavor meals that are ready to nourish your family inside and out. Whether you're Keto, gluten-free or just trying to eat a tiny bit better than before, this book is for you. Whether you are cooking for a big family or just for yourself, this book is for you. In these pages you'll find the yummiest food, made simple and easy.

I think it's safe to say that I'm used to cooking with the clock ticking—just ask Gordon Ramsay. Sure, during my two stints on *MasterChef* I had to cook some pretty complicated dishes in a short amount of time. But when the clock is ticking, you're forced to think about how to get the most flavor out of ingredients very quickly. And that's exactly what I did in this book too. I'm bringing you big flavors and bold answers to the question, "What's for dinner?"

As a food lover and chef, I spend all day and night around food—it's my world. But in the past, that led me to develop a pretty unhealthy relationship with the food around me. So I had to make a change. I lost over 80 pounds in one year, and I did it by eating my way to health, not dieting. I found a way to make chef-worthy meals at home that were so good, you'd forget they were "healthy." And I believe that's the key to success on any diet, Keto or otherwise. You need to love the food you're eating. Period. So I set out on a mission to share the food I was creating. To show that you can eat better and feel better without suffering through a diet. So the recipes in this book are good for anyone—Keto or not. It's just good food. It's food without unnecessary sugars or flours. Food your kids will love. Food your spouse will ask for again and again. Dinners you can add to your weekly menu that are quick, cheap and easy to make, even after a long work day. And honestly, these are recipes that will bring out your inner master chef too.

Throughout the book, I've included pro tips, tricks and bonus recipes to help you be the best cook you can be, all while using only common grocery-store ingredients. The food in this book is approachable, but with a chef's kiss. So, what are you waiting for? Put on your apron, and let's get cooking!

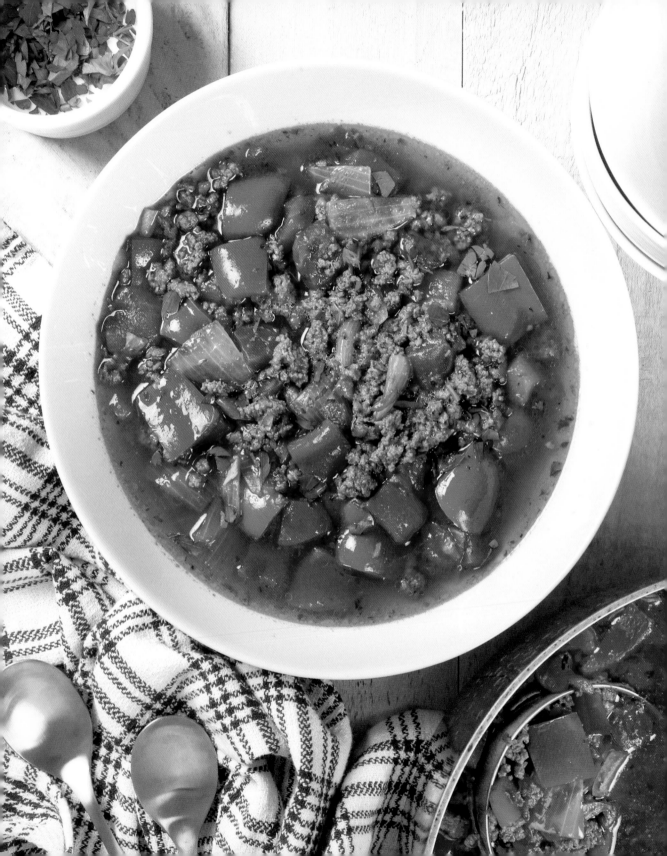

deciding what's for dinner

You'll notice that every recipe in this book includes some valuable information to help you decide what's for dinner. As always, I've included the macros (nutritional content) for each recipe. But I've also included more information about each dish, like the cooking times and quick reference icons for dietary restrictions and allergies—see below for an explanation. Please note that all the recipes in this book are sugar-free and Keto-friendly as well.

It's a Piece of Cake!

Every—and I mean every—recipe in this book is designed to be super quick and easy. In fact, I'd say they're all a piece of cake! But some nights you might be feeling "chefy-er" than other nights, so I've provided a quick way to identify the easiest of the easy recipes. And when you're ready to impress with slightly more ambitious recipes, I've got you covered there too.

 1 Piece of Cake

Extremely easy with minimal cutting and steps involved

 2 Pieces of Cake

Quick and easy, but with light knife work and cooking steps required

 3 Pieces of Cake

Slightly more involved recipes with multiple steps, which yield extra impressive results

Dietary Quick Guide

 Dairy-free   Gluten-free   Soy-free

 Dairy-optional   Nut-free Vegetarian

Macros

I've included the macro-nutrition facts for every recipe in this book. Depending on your exact goals and dietary needs, the macros can help guide you toward recipes that best fit your lifestyle. Please note that the macros are based on one serving, and do not include any optional ingredients listed. Also keep in mind that macros can vary quite dramatically based on the exact brands of each ingredient you use and the size of your produce, so shop wisely and check those labels when you're shopping.

Tips, Tricks, and More!

Make sure to check out the Chef's Cheat Sheet chapter (page 146) for everything from pantry basics to time- and money-saving tips and tricks to help you plan and cook your best meals.

Active vs. Total Cooking Times

The "total time" on a recipe is the estimated time it will take you to make that dish from start to finish. Whereas the "active cooking times" only include the time you'll actually be in the kitchen preparing the food. For instance, if something is baking in the oven for 15 minutes, that would not be a part of the active cooking time.

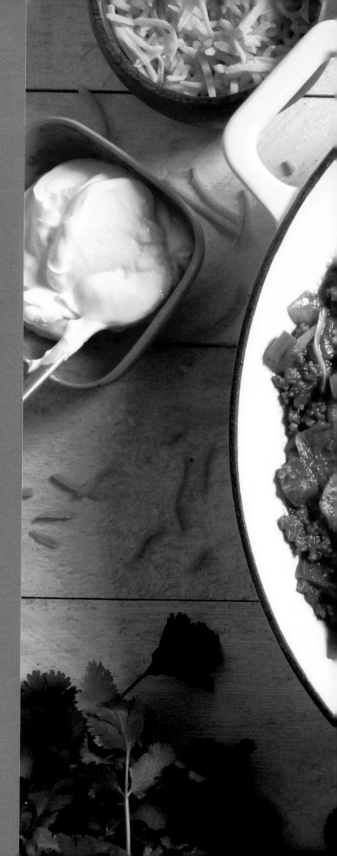

brisk beef

Beef is the best, and you can't convince me otherwise. I mean, what's better than a perfectly juicy steak? Or a burger? Nothing. Absolutely nothing. So naturally, I had to start this book off right—with nothing but the best beef recipes on the planet! Here are some damn good dinners you can make in 30 minutes or less.

Texas Chili-Rubbed Ribeye with Fiery Chipotle Butter (page 14)

Bacon Cheeseburger Skillet with "Big Mike" Sauce (page 17)

Mouthwatering Mongolian Beef (page 18)

15-Minute Heavenly Steak Bites (page 21)

No-Frilly Weeknight Chili (page 22)

Thousand Island Reuben Skillet (page 25)

Finger-Lickin' Low-Carb Steak Tacos with Smoky Crema (page 26)

Mellow Mushroom Smothered Tri-Tips (page 29)

Keto Korean Barbecue Short Ribs (L.A. Galbi) (page 30)

Blue Cheese Lovers' Steak and Asparagus Sauté (page 33)

Mediterranean-Spiced Kebabs with Dill Yogurt Drizzle (page 34)

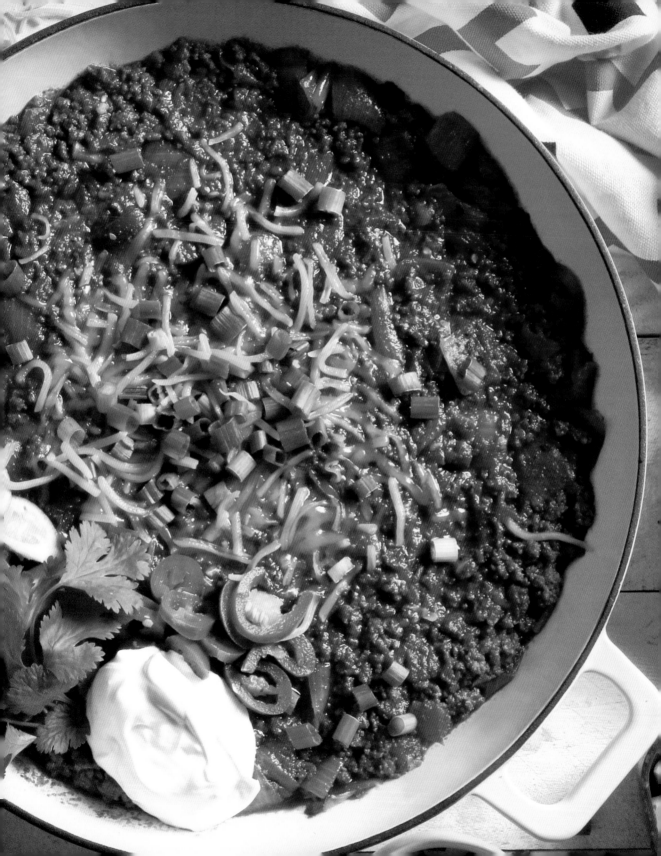

active cooking time
25 minutes

total time
30 minutes

macros per serving

calories
969

protein
60.2 g

fat
85.6 g

net carbs
0.6 g

texas chili-rubbed ribeye with fiery chipotle butter

This beefy dinner is full of big flavors and an even bigger attitude. This is a spicy chili-crusted, juicy steak topped with a sexy and smoky chipotle-infused compound butter. Giddyap, cowboy! It's time to bring the wild west into your kitchen.

Try pairing this with the Herby Pan-Roasted Mushrooms on page 126.

fiery chipotle butter

3 tbsp (42 g) salted Irish-style butter

⅛ tsp sea salt

½ tbsp packed chopped fresh cilantro

1 clove garlic, finely grated or minced

1 tsp minced chipotle peppers in adobo sauce (from a 3.5-oz [99-g] can; add more if you like it extra spicy)

chili-rubbed ribeye

1 tsp chipotle powder (for spicy) or smoked paprika (for mild)

1 tsp chili powder

1 tsp sea salt

2 tsp (4 g) freshly cracked black pepper

2 (16-oz [454-g]) bone-in ribeye steaks

1 tbsp (15 ml) avocado oil

2 sprigs fresh rosemary

Take the butter out of the fridge at least an hour ahead of time, so it softens completely. Optionally microwave the butter on the low (10 percent power) setting in 30-second increments until the butter soft, but not melted. Take the steaks out of the fridge about 15 minutes ahead to temper.

To make the butter, add to a small bowl the butter, salt, cilantro, garlic and chipotle peppers. With spoon, mash everything together until mixed completely. Stretch out a long piece of plastic wrap o your countertop. Spoon the butter right in the center of the plastic wrap, then fold the wrap lengthwise over the butter, sealing the edges together. Using your hands, roll and mold the butter into a log shape making sure there are no air bubbles in the plastic as you roll. Twist the ends of the wrap tightly, the place it in the freezer to set.

To make the steaks, warm a large (12-inch [30-cm]) cast-iron skillet over medium heat. In a small bowl mix together the chipotle powder, chili powder, salt and black pepper, then coat the steaks on all side with the spice blend (just under 1 tablespoon [6 g] of spice blend per steak). Once the pan is hot, add the avocado oil and place the steaks in the pan. Add the rosemary sprigs around the steak. Without moving the steaks, let them sear for 5 minutes, then flip and sear for 3 to 4 minutes, or just until you've reached your desired internal temperature. *Note: The exact cooking time really depends on the thickness of the steak, so using a meat thermometer is the best way to ensure a perfect cook. See the Meat Temperature Guide on page 157.* Take the steaks out of the pan, and let them rest on a cooling rack for 5 minutes When you're ready to serve, plate the steaks with a generous slice of the compound butter on top.

pro tip: Are you ready for a barbecue? This steak is delicious on the grill too. Also, you can use the simple chili rub in this recipe on just about anything. Try it on ribs, burgers, wings, pork chops or even fish. And don't waste the leftover chipotle peppers—check out the Finger-Lickin' Low-Carb Steak Tacos with Smoky Crema on page 26.

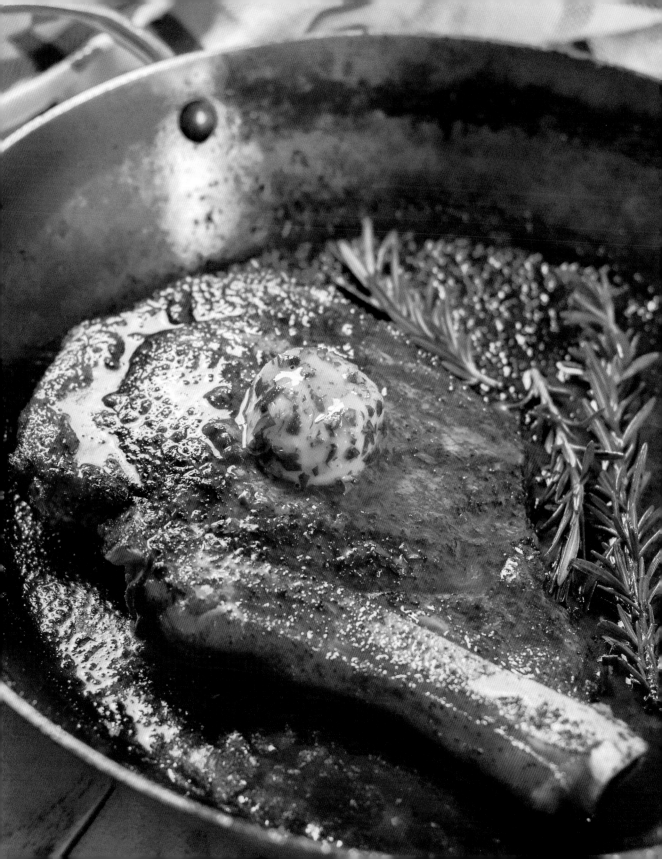

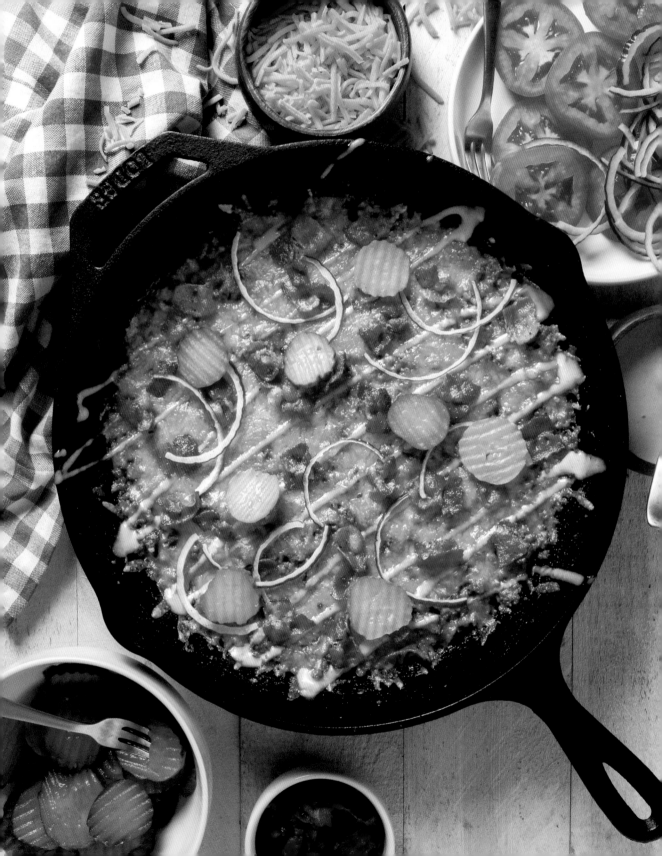

bacon cheeseburger skillet with "big mike" sauce

Out of all the recipes in this book, this is probably the dish I make most often (at least once a week). Sure, it's "just" ground beef, but something special happens here. You close your eyes, take a bite and are somehow transported right to the drive-thru line—and I mean that in the best way possible. It really does taste like the fast-food classic. You can make this in 20 minutes too, which is quicker than the actual drive-thru line anyway. And it's much, much healthier and more nutritious. So skip the line, save the money and make this instead.

serves
6

active cooking time
20 minutes

total time
20 minutes

macros per serving

calories
608

protein
37 g

fat
47 g

net carbs
2.8 g

cheeseburger skillet

- oz (170 g) no-sugar bacon, cut into " (2.5-cm) pieces
- lb (907 g) 90-percent lean ground beef
- tsp sea salt
- tsp freshly cracked black pepper
- tsp (12 g) seasoning salt
- tsp garlic powder
- tsp onion powder
- tsp (10 ml) Worcestershire sauce
- ½ cups (170 g) shredded Cheddar cheese
- white or red onion, thinly sliced

"big mike" sauce

- ½ cup (120 ml) mayonnaise
- 2 tbsp (30 ml) no-sugar ketchup
- 1 tsp apple cider vinegar
- 1 tsp Worcestershire sauce
- ¼ tsp sea salt
- 1 tsp onion powder
- 1 tsp granulated sweetener (I recommend allulose)

Pickles, sliced onions, pickled jalapeños, sliced avocado or sliced tomato, to serve (optional)

To make the skillet, using a large (12-inch [30-cm]) cast-iron or oven-safe skillet over medium-high heat, fry the bacon for 5 to 6 minutes, or until it is crispy. Take the bacon out of the pan and set it aside.

Turn the heat up to high and add the ground beef to the pan with the remaining bacon fat. Break up the meat with a spatula, then stir in the sea salt, black pepper, seasoning salt, garlic powder, onion powder and Worcestershire sauce. Sauté for 4 minutes, or until the meat is browned and cooked through.

While the meat cooks, set the oven to broil. Use the back of a spatula to press the ground beef in one flat, even layer. Carefully pour out any excess grease and then top it evenly with the cheese and onion. Place the skillet in the oven and broil for 2 to 3 minutes, or until the cheese is fully melted and bubbly.

To make the sauce, in a small bowl, mix the mayonnaise, ketchup, apple cider vinegar, Worcestershire, salt, onion powder and sweetener. When the skillet is finished, take it out of the oven and drizzle it with the sauce. Then, top it with the crispy bacon and any of your favorite toppings. Serve family style and dig right in!

pro tip: Have fun with the flavors in this dish! Love a good mushroom and Swiss burger? Replace the Cheddar with Swiss and add sautéed mushrooms. I've even topped this with a little marinara, mozzarella and pepperoni slices for a pizza burger skillet! The possibilities are endless.

serves
3

active cooking time
25 minutes

total time
25 minutes

macros per serving

calories
524

protein
55 g

fat
30.5 g

net carbs
8.3 g

mouthwatering mongolian beef

Mongolian beef is definitely not from Mongolia, but I can't seem to pinpoint exactl where it originates from. Most theories have it born in Chinese restaurants here in th U.S. All I know is, it's undeniably delicious. And it's not typically made as sweet as man other Chinese-American classics, so making this sugar-free version was really seamless What I love most about this dish is the almost crazy amount of scallions in it. I can't thin of many other dishes anywhere that use this many scallions, and it's so wonderful to se this humble allium featured. So yeah, this may seem like a lot of scallions, but trust me that's the point! Sweet, salty and packed with umami savoriness, this is the dish I crav basically every night.

Try pairing this with the Easy Egg Drop Soup on page 99.

1½ lb (680 g) flank steak (see Pro Tip)

8 scallions, root ends trimmed

¼ cup (60 ml) avocado oil

2 tsp (6 g) minced or grated fresh ginger

6 cloves garlic, minced

1 tsp crushed red pepper flakes or Chinese dried red chili peppers

½ cup (120 ml) low-sodium soy sauce

2 tbsp (18 g) brown sweetener (I recommend Swerve brand)

Slice the steak very thinly—the thinner the better (see Pro Tip). Make sure to slice perpendicular to, c "against," the grain, then set the steak aside. Slice the scallions into 2-inch (5-cm) pieces, separatin the lighter green ends from the darker ends, and set them aside.

Place a large wok or skillet (12 inches [30 cm] or larger) over high heat and add the avocado oi Once the oil is very hot, add the sliced beef, stirring constantly, and stir-fry for 4 minutes, or until th edges of the meat become slightly browned. *Note: This may seem like you're overcooking the bee but this will be the one time I encourage you to cook your beef toward well-done, to help make th beef crispier *wink*.* Use a slotted spoon or tongs to take the beef out of the wok, leaving the o behind, and set the beef aside on a plate.

Add the ginger, garlic and red pepper flakes to the wok, and stir-fry for 30 seconds. Add the soy sauc and sweetener, and simmer for 3 minutes, or until the sauce starts to thicken. Place the beef back int the wok, along with the lighter/white scallion ends, and stir-fry for 3 minutes, or until all the liquid ha evaporated from the pan and the sauce is sticking to the beef. Turn off the heat and stir in the gree scallion tops. Pour the Mongolian beef onto a large plate and serve family-style while it's steaming ho

pro tip: A nice trick for cutting the steak extra thin is placing it in the freezer for 5 to 10 minutes before you slice. This will firm up the meat and make it easier to cut into thin slices.

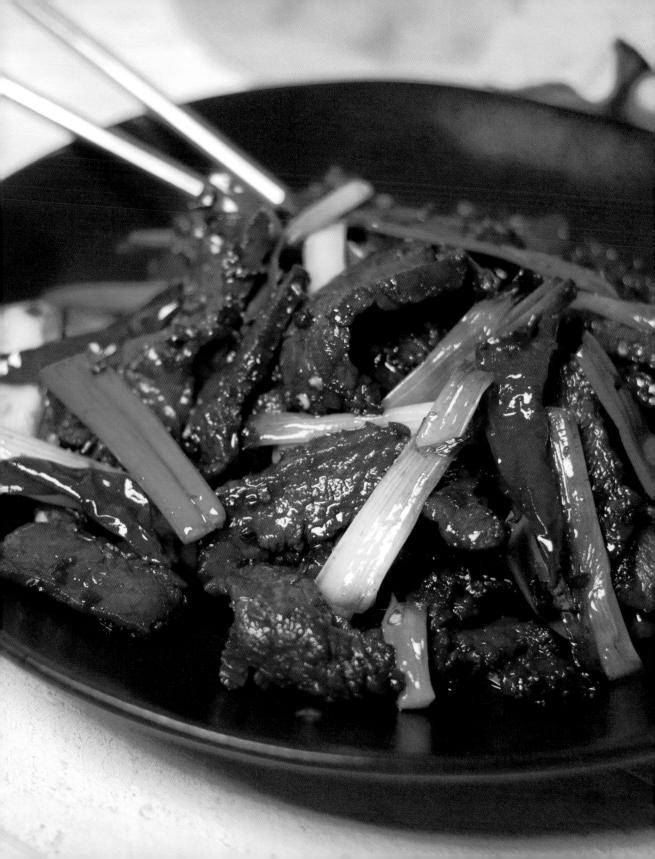

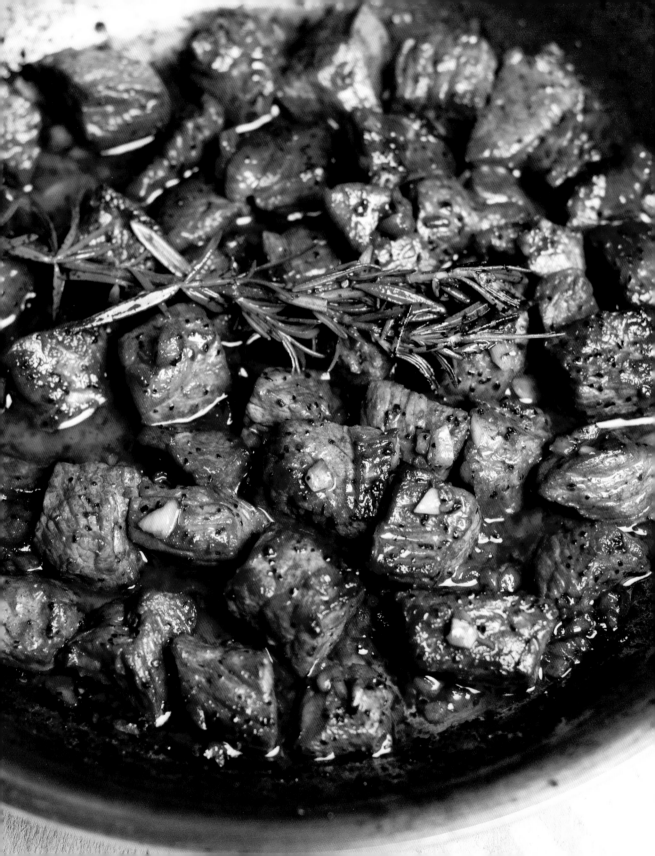

5-minute heavenly steak bites

When I call this *heavenly*, I mean it—this dish is pure indulgence. One bite, and you'll wish you doubled the recipe. Sure, it's a lot of butter . . . but it's worth it! In fact, I suggest buying a high-quality Irish-style or grass-fed butter for this. Grass-fed butter is loaded with healthy fats and has much more flavor than your standard butter, so this is one occasion where it's really worth the extra cost. And because this dish is super low-carb, treat yourself to one of the most delicious meals ever. Just don't hold back on the garlic (and make sure you have mints nearby).

Try pairing this with the Cheesy Baked Asparagus on page 118.

Try pairing this with the Cheesy Baked Asparagus on page 118.

1 lb (454 g) top sirloin steak (see Pro Tip)

1 tbsp (15 ml) avocado oil

½ tsp sea salt

½ tsp freshly cracked black pepper

¼ cup (57 g) salted Irish-style butter

6 cloves garlic, minced

1 sprig fresh rosemary

1 tbsp (6 g) grated Parmesan cheese

Cut the steak into ½-inch (1.3-cm) cubes, removing any large pieces of fat. Place a large (12-inch [30-cm]) skillet over high heat and add the avocado oil. Meanwhile, toss the steak bites in the salt and pepper until evenly coated. When the oil is smoking hot, place the steak bites into the oil in an even layer. Without moving them, let the steak sear for 1 minute on the first side. Flip over each piece individually to another side with tongs, and sear for 1 minute. Repeat this step on a third side, until the total cooking time has been 3 minutes, and your steak bites have some noticeable brown edges. *Note: If you're making a double batch of this, you still want to sear the steak in two batches to ensure proper browning of the meat.*

Take the bites out of the pan and set them aside to rest. Place the same pan back over medium heat and add the butter. As soon as the butter is mostly melted, add the minced garlic and rosemary sprig. Let the garlic sauté for 2 minutes, or until it's just turning golden. Turn off the heat and put the steak bites back into the pan, along with the Parmesan. Toss everything together and serve family-style in the pan while it's hot and bubbly.

pro tip: It's tough to make this recipe any more delectable, but for a real treat, try making this with filet mignon instead of sirloin. The filet will be incredibly tender and luxurious . . . sounds like a date night to me!

serves
2

active cooking time
15 minutes

total time
15 minutes

macros per serving

calories
743

protein
47.6 g

fat
58.8 g

net carbs
2.9 g

serves
4

active cooking time
20 minutes

total time
30 minutes

macros per serving

calories
580

protein
43.9 g

fat
35.6 g

net carbs
8.5 g

no-frilly weeknight chili

When I think of chili, I think of hours standing in front of the stove, nursing the chili t perfection. But some nights, I just want chili without all that effort. This is a pared-dow version of a classic chili that still packs in all the flavor and heat you expect from th slow-cooked version. And in true Texas style, it has no beans, which also means it's low carb too. So there's no excuse not to make this deliciously comforting recipe—cheap quick, tasty and healthy. What more could you ask for?

Try pairing this with the Fab 5-Minute Spanish Rice on page 125.

1 tbsp (15 ml) avocado oil
1 yellow onion, chopped
1–2 jalapeños, chopped
2 lb (907 g) 85-percent lean ground beef
¼ cup (66 g) tomato paste
1 tsp sea salt
1 tsp freshly cracked black pepper
2 tbsp (13 g) chili powder
2 tbsp (14 g) paprika
1 tbsp (8 g) cumin

1 tbsp (8 g) garlic powder
1 tbsp (7 g) onion powder
½–1 tsp cayenne (optional)
2 (10-oz [283-g]) cans fire-roasted diced tomatoes and green chiles, drained (I recommen Rotel brand)
1 cup (240 ml) beef broth

Shredded Cheddar, sour cream, sliced scallions and/or pickled jalapeños, to serve (optional)

Warm a large Dutch oven or lidded pot over high heat. Add the avocado oil, onion and jalapeño and sauté for 2 minutes, or until the veggies start to soften and brown. Add the beef and break it u into small pieces. After 2 minutes, add the tomato paste, salt, black pepper, chili powder, paprika cumin, garlic powder, onion powder and cayenne (if using), and mix well to combine with the mec and veggies. Sauté for 1 minute, then stir in the canned tomatoes and broth. Put the lid on the po leaving it slightly open to let steam escape. Lower the heat to medium-low and simmer for 10 minutes Serve the chili divided into four bowls or serve family-style with any of your favorite toppings. I love m chili topped with Cheddar, scallions and sour cream.

pro tip: Try making this in a slow cooker! Simply add all the ingredients in the cooker and cook on high for 4 hours or low for 8 hours.

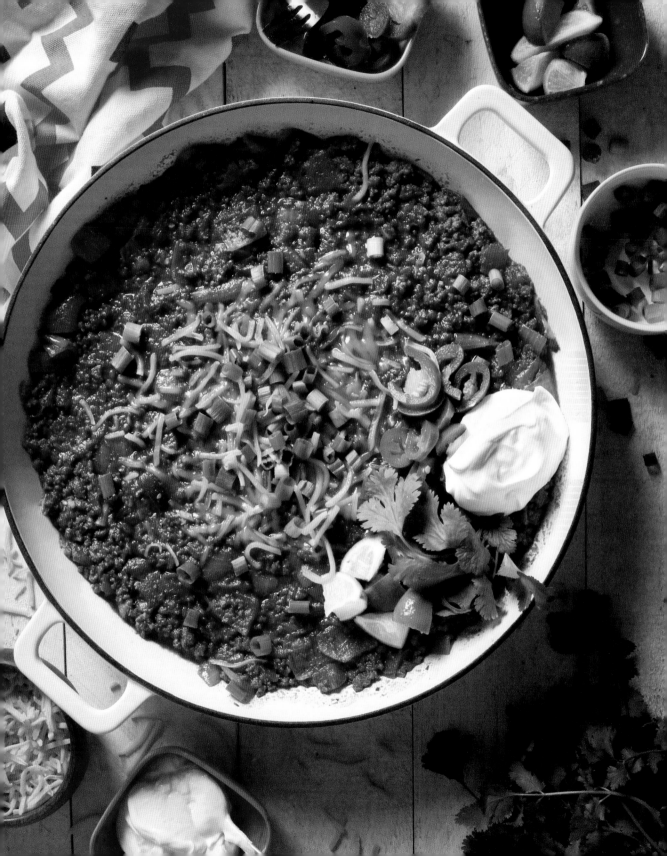

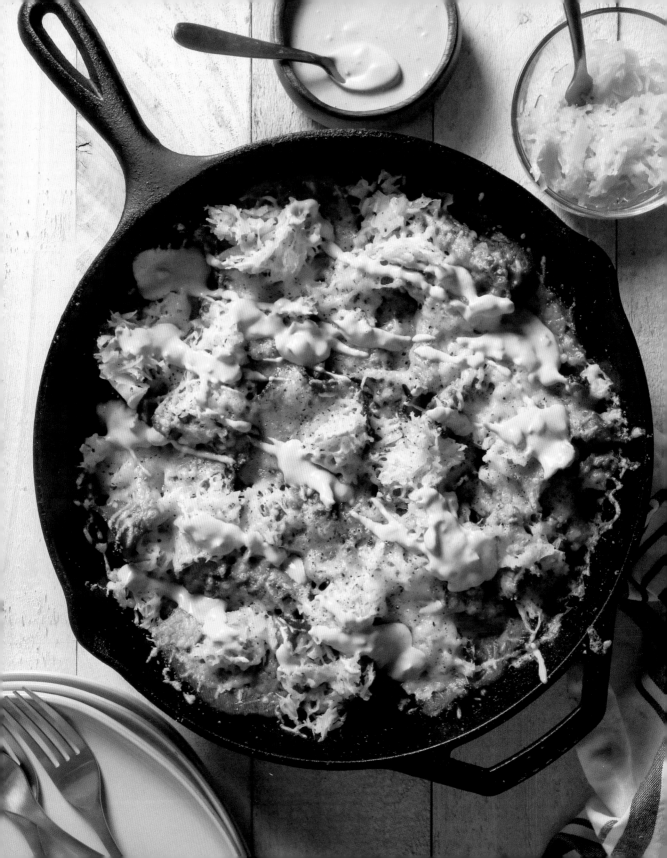

thousand island reuben skillet

This recipe brings the New York deli right to your kitchen! Cheesy, creamy and packed with protein, this awesome dinner can be made in just 15 minutes. The best part is that there is no cutting, slicing or prep work, so it's great for a quick weeknight meal. You can also customize this to make it your own. Try using turkey pastrami to make this a Rachel skillet. Don't like sauerkraut? Just leave it out or try topping it with coleslaw instead. I also recommend doubling the Thousand Island dressing recipe and storing the leftovers in your refrigerator in a jar or squeeze bottle. It's a great sugar-free dressing to keep on-hand for your salads and sandwiches, and it'll last about 10 days in your fridge.

Try pairing this with the Herby Pan-Roasted Mushrooms on page 126.

Try pairing this with the Herby Pan-Roasted Mushrooms on page 126.

thousand island dressing

½ cup (120 ml) mayonnaise

3 tbsp (45 ml) no-sugar ketchup

1 tbsp (15 ml) fresh lemon juice (from ½ lemon)

1 tbsp (15 ml) dill relish

reuben skillet

1 tbsp (15 ml) avocado oil

1½ lb (680 g) sliced pastrami or corned beef (see Pro Tip)

1 tsp freshly cracked black pepper, plus extra for garnish

1 cup (150 g) drained sauerkraut

4 oz (113 g) shredded or sliced Swiss cheese

Set the oven to broil.

To make the dressing, in a medium bowl, add the mayonnaise, ketchup, lemon juice and relish, and mix very well to combine. Set it aside in the fridge.

To make the skillet, place a large (12-inch [30-cm]) cast-iron or oven-safe skillet over medium heat and add the avocado oil. Once hot, add the pastrami and black pepper, and sauté for 2 to 3 minutes, or until the meat just starts to lightly brown and warm through. Top the pastrami evenly with the sauerkraut and cheese. Place the skillet into the oven to broil for 2 to 3 minutes, or just until the cheese is melted and bubbly. Take the skillet out of the oven, top with extra black pepper (if using) and drizzle the dressing on top. Enjoy family-style, served with any leftover sauce on the side.

pro tip: If you're using corned beef, remember that it is the star of this recipe, so it's worth splurging on the good stuff from the deli counter. But, for a more budget-friendly option, you can absolutely make this with deli turkey, roast beef or even seasoned ground beef instead. If you're using ground beef, sauté it in the pan first with salt and pepper until it's cooked through before topping it with the sauerkraut and cheese.

serves
4

active cooking time
15 minutes

total time
15 minutes

macros per serving

calories
494

protein
34.7 g

fat
37.1 g

net carbs
5.3 g

serves
3

active cooking time
30 minutes

total time
30 minutes

macros per serving

calories
597

protein
48.6 g

fat
35.9 g

net carbs
8.2 g

finger-lickin' low-carb steak tacos with smoky crema

Here in Texas, we *live* for tacos. So naturally, I had to bring you some real-deal bee tacos—no crunchy taco shells, no ground beef, no taco seasoning. Instead, these taco are filled with the juiciest marinated skirt steak you can imagine and loaded with you favorite toppings. This is how you elevate your next Taco Tuesday . . . Texas style!

Try pairing this with the Fab 5-Minute Spanish Rice on page 125.

for the skirt steak tacos
½ tsp sea salt
½ tsp freshly cracked black pepper
½ tsp garlic powder
½ tsp chipotle powder (for spicy) or smoked paprika (for mild)
½ tsp cumin
1 lb (454 g) skirt steak
2 tbsp (30 ml) avocado oil, divided
6 small (taco-sized) low-carb tortillas

for the smoky chipotle crema
½ cup (120 ml) sour cream
1½ tbsp (22 ml) adobo sauce (from a 3.5-oz [99-g] can of chipotle peppers in adobo sauce; see **Pro Tip**)
1 tbsp (15 ml) fresh lime juice (from 1 lime)

Sliced avocado, lime wedges, cilantro, pico de gallo and/or cotija cheese, for serving (optional

To make the tacos, in a small bowl, add the salt, black pepper, garlic powder, chipotle powder c smoked paprika and cumin, and mix until the spice blend is uniform. Place the steak on a cutting boar and use a sharp knife to very carefully trim off any of the excess silverskin or fat on either side of the ski steak—this will help ensure that the steak is nice and tender. Rub 1 tablespoon (15 ml) of the avocad oil onto the steak, and evenly coat all sides with the spice blend.

Warm a large (12-inch [30-cm]) skillet or griddle pan over medium heat. Once hot, coat the pan wit the remaining avocado oil, then sear the steak for 4 minutes on each side (for medium-rare). Once the steak is done, set it aside on a cooling rack or plate to rest for 5 minutes.

While the steak rests, make the sauce by mixing together the sour cream, adobo sauce and lime juice in a small bowl. Set the sauce aside, then get all the rest of your favorite taco toppings together—I like mine with avocado slices, cotija cheese and lime wedges. It's fun to serve these tacos by setting up c "make-your-own taco bar," with all the sides and add-ins in separate bowls. Then warm the tortillas b lightly toasting them in a dry pan over medium-high heat for about 10 seconds on each side, and se them on a plate. Dice the steak into small ½-inch (1.3-cm) cubes, and serve along with the tortillas crema and taco toppings of your choosing.

pro tip: Don't waste the leftover chipotles in the can from this recipe. Use them in the Texas Chile-Rubbed Ribeye with Fiery Chipotle Butter on page 14, or chop up two or three and add them to the No-Frilly Weeknight Chili (page 22) for an added punch of flavor. Or you can double or triple the smoky crema recipe and store it in a sealed jar in the fridge for up to 10 days. Spread it on your next burger for a tasty treat.

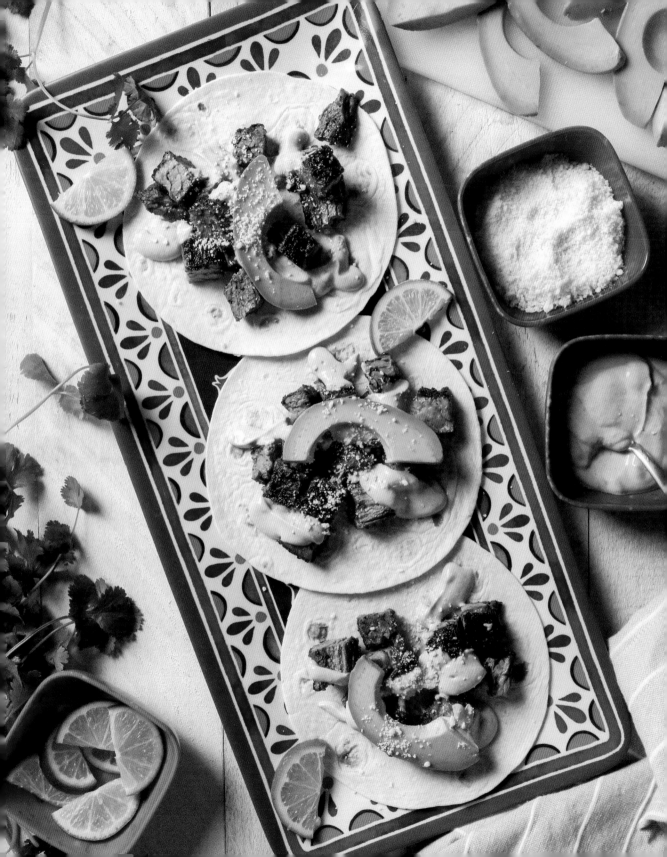

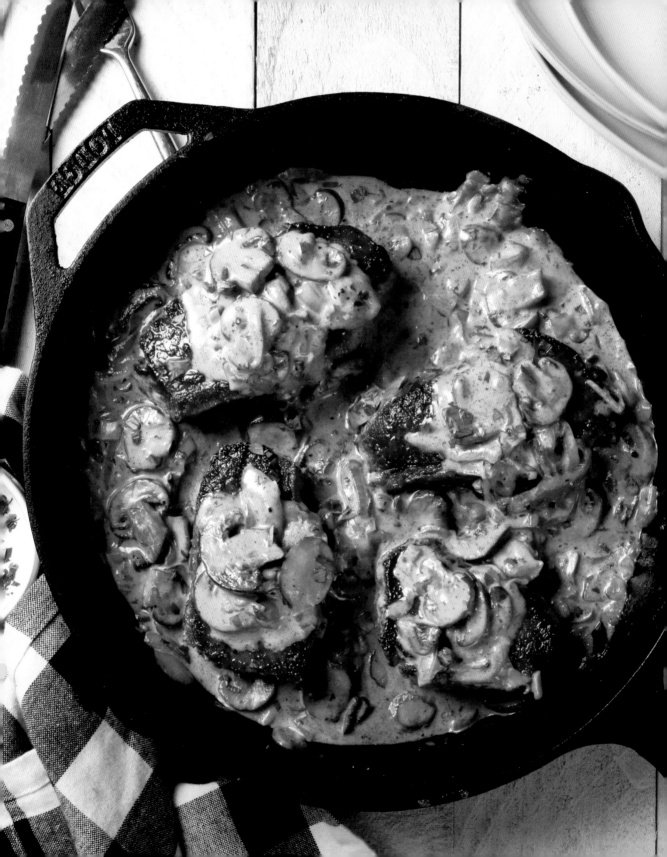

mellow mushroom smothered tri-tips

oes this recipe use magical mushrooms? No. But this dish is so good, you'll be tripping
ut! Juicy steaks covered in sautéed mushrooms, onions and a deliciously creamy
ravy? Now *that* sounds like a good trip to me! This recipe is rich and comforting and
rprisingly easy to make. So mellow out, dude! We got your dinner plans covered.

y pairing this with the Sweet Balsamic-Glazed Brussels on page 121.

serves
4

active cooking time
30 minutes

total time
30 minutes

macros per serving

calories
484

protein
48.4 g

fat
30.5 g

net carbs
2.8 g

---

lb (907 g) tri-tip steaks (see Pro Tip)

tbsp (15 ml) avocado oil

½ tsp (9 g) sea salt, divided

½ tsp (3 g) freshly cracked black pepper,
vided

yellow onion, thinly sliced

cloves garlic, thinly sliced

8 oz (226 g) pre-sliced baby bella (cremini)
mushrooms

1 cup (240 ml) beef broth

¼ cup (60 ml) heavy cream or half-and-half
(coconut cream for dairy-free)

¼ tsp xanthan gum (for thickening, optional)

1 tbsp (4 g) chopped fresh parsley, divided

ke the steaks out of the fridge about 15 minutes ahead to temper. Heat a large (12-inch
0-cm]) skillet over medium-high heat and add the avocado oil. Season each side of the steaks with
teaspoon of salt and ¼ teaspoon of black pepper. Once the pan is smoking hot, sear the steaks
r 4 minutes on each side, or until the steaks have a dark brown crust. Then, sear the edges of each
eak for 30 seconds per side to get an all-around crust. *Note: For a perfect cook on your steak, check*
e internal temperature of each steak using a meat thermometer—see the Meat Temperature Guide on
age 157. Once cooked, take the steaks out of the pan and set them aside on a plate or cooling rack
rest while you make the sauce.

ace the same pan over medium-low heat and add the onion and garlic. Sauté for 2 minutes, stirring
onstantly. Add the mushrooms and the remaining salt and pepper, and sauté for 2 minutes. Just as the
ushrooms start to get some color and soften, pour in the beef broth and heavy cream. Bring the sauce
a boil, and let the veggies simmer for 2 minutes, or until the mushrooms are fully cooked. If using,
rinkle the xanthan gum into the sauce and stir until the sauce gets thicker, like a light gravy. Turn off
e heat and stir in half of the chopped parsley. Nestle the steaks back into the sauce, spooning the
elicious gravy all over the top. Garnish with the remaining parsley and serve family-style.

pro tip: Tri-tip is a wonderful and often overlooked cut of beef. But this recipe works
well with almost any cut of steak, including New York strip, sirloin, T-bone or ribeye. On
a budget? Try this with cube steak. Heck, you can even make this with pork chops or
chicken thighs! For a luxurious upgrade, melt Swiss cheese, Gruyère or even blue cheese
on top of the smothered steaks.

serves
3

active cooking time
20 minutes

total time
25 minutes

macros per serving

calories
489

protein
40.9 g

fat
32.4 g

net carbs
5.5 g

keto korean barbecue short ribs (l.a. galbi)

I was lucky enough to spend some time in South Korea many years ago, and to this da it remains one of my most treasured culinary inspirations. I'll never forget my genuin amazement at every single bite of food I encountered, or what I learned there. C course, Korean barbecue has become quite ubiquitous here in the U.S.—and for goo reason: it's delicious! At Korean restaurants, *galbi* (ribs, in Korean) is *essential* to an KBBQ menu. But L.A. galbi was actually developed in Los Angeles by Korean immigran and has since made its way back to Korea. The crosscut (also known as flanken cut) sho ribs are tender and quick to marinate. Although pear would be traditionally added t this marinade, I left it out, along with the sugar, to keep this recipe low-carb. But this perhaps one of my all-time favorite dishes, and it just so happens to be quick, health and super fun to make.

¼ white or yellow onion

2 cloves garlic

1 tsp minced or grated fresh ginger

¼ tsp freshly cracked black pepper

2 tbsp (18 g) brown sweetener (I recommend Swerve brand) or light brown sugar (28 g)

⅓ cup (80 ml) low-sodium soy sauce

2 tbsp (30 ml) rice wine vinegar

1 tbsp (15 ml) sesame oil

2 lb (907 g) bone-in, crosscut (flanken cut) beef short ribs (see Pro Tip)

1 tbsp (15 ml) avocado oil

1 tsp sesame seeds

2 scallions, sliced

Green leaf lettuce, rice or rice substitute, ssamjang (Korean soybean paste) for dipping and/or kimchi, for serving (optional)

Use a microplane or small grater to grate the onion, garlic and ginger. If you don't have a grater, ju mince everything with a knife until it's almost a fine paste. In a medium bowl or large ziplock bag, ad the onion, garlic, ginger, pepper, sweetener, soy sauce, vinegar and sesame oil. Toss the short rib into the sauce, coating them completely. Let them marinate for a minimum of 5 minutes, but you ca also make this a day ahead and let the meat marinate overnight to get even more flavor—the longe the better.

Warm a large (12-inch [30-cm]) skillet or grill pan (you can also do this on an outdoor grill) ove medium-high heat. Grease the pan with the avocado oil. Once the pan is very hot, place the ribs dow flat and sear them for 2 minutes, or until you get a nice char. Repeat on the other side for 2 minute You may need to sear the short ribs in two batches, depending on the size of the pan. Take the rib out of the pan and set them on a plate. Sprinkle the tops with the sesame seeds and scallions. Serv with your favorite sides.

pro tip: Most grocery stores now stock flanken-cut short ribs, but if you can't find them, try asking the butcher at the meat department counter. They may be able to cut it for you—it never hurts to ask. Also, almost any Asian supermarket should stock them. If you still can't find them, any thin-sliced beef will work for this recipe.

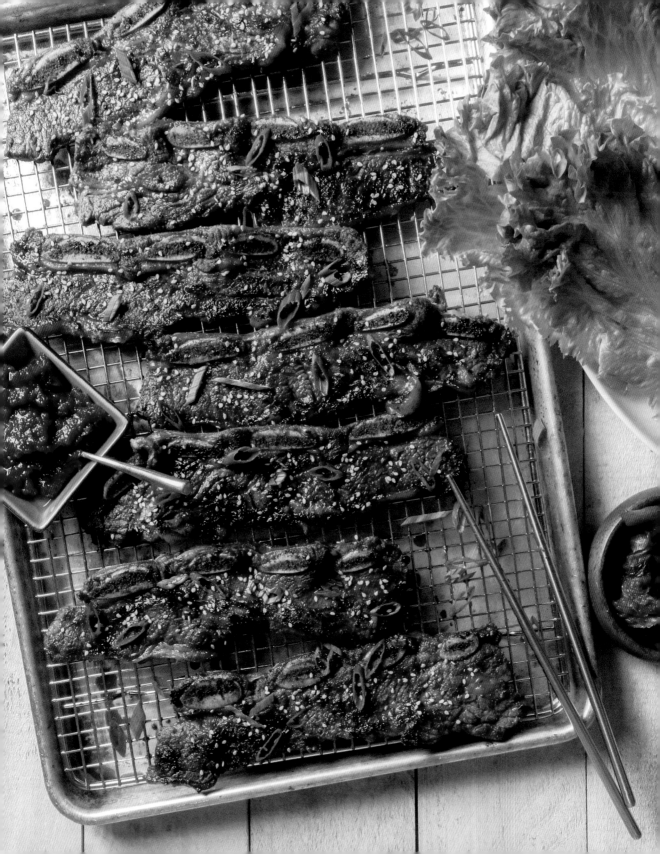

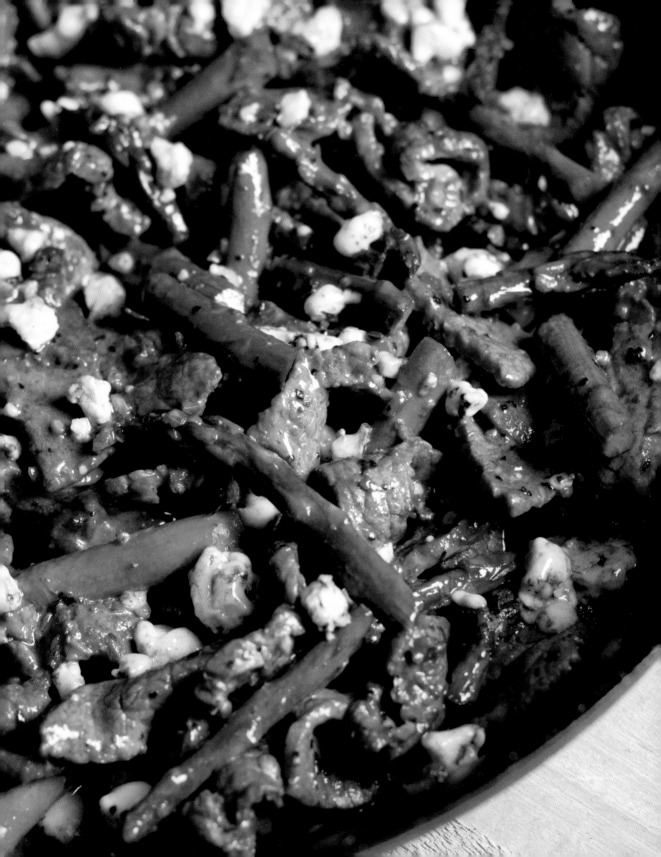

blue cheese lovers' steak and asparagus sauté

If you are reading this right now, you're probably a blue cheese lover. (It's safe to assume everyone else was too scared to even open this page. But that is their loss!) For us blue cheese fans, this is the recipe we've always wanted. And it's unapologetically blue cheesy—and I say that proudly! This is tender steak, coated in a blue cheese sauce and sprinkled with even more blue cheese melted on top. It's sheer luxury made easy; a full steak house dinner, simplified into a perfect one-pot meal. And did I mention you can make it in 20 minutes?

Try pairing this with the *Sweet Balsamic-Glazed Brussels* on page 121.

serves
4

active cooking time
20 minutes

total time
20 minutes

macros per serving

calories
636

protein
59.8 g

fat
40.5 g

net carbs
4.8 g

1 lb (454 g) asparagus

2 lb (907 g) thin-sliced top round/eye of round steak (see Pro Tip)

2 tbsp (30 ml) avocado oil

2 tbsp (18 g) Montreal steak seasoning (I recommend McCormick brand)

2 tbsp (28 g) unsalted butter

4 cloves garlic, minced

1 tbsp (15 ml) Worcestershire sauce

1 tbsp (15 ml) balsamic vinegar

4 oz (113 g) crumbled blue cheese, divided

Prepare the asparagus by cutting off the bottom inch (2.5 cm) or so to remove the fibrous ends. Then, slice the asparagus into 1-inch (2.5-cm) pieces. (For presentation, I like to cut the asparagus on an angle.) Set them aside on a plate. If you're using pre-sliced steak from the meat department, simply cut those into smaller bite-sized pieces. If you're using a whole steak, slice it as thin as you can. (See Pro Tip.)

Place a large (12-inch [30-cm]) skillet over high heat and add the avocado oil. While it's warming up, sprinkle the steak seasoning on the beef until evenly coated. Once the oil is smoking hot, add the steak and sear for 3 minutes, or just until the steak is cooked through. Be sure to stir the meat halfway through. Take the beef out of the pan and set it aside on a plate to rest, leaving all the liquid in the pan. To the pan, stir in the butter, garlic, Worcestershire sauce and balsamic. As soon as the butter is melted, add the cut asparagus and sauté for 2 minutes. Stir 2 ounces (57 g) of the blue cheese into the mixture, until it starts to melt into the sauce. Place the beef back into the pan and toss it in the sauce, cooking for 1 minute. Turn off the heat, top with the remaining blue cheese and serve family-style.

pro tip: Can't find the pre-sliced steak? Buy any of your favorite steaks (e.g. ribeye, tri-tip, round or flank) and slice them as thinly as you can. A nice trick for cutting the steak extra thin is placing it in the freezer for 5 to 10 minutes before you slice. This will firm up the meat and make it easier to cut. For an extra boost of flavor, add 8 ounces (226 g) of sliced portobello or cremini mushrooms along with the asparagus.

brisk beef

mediterranean-spiced kebabs with dill yogurt drizzle

This all-in-one meal is perfect for when you really want to "spice" things up for dinner. Although, to be clear, these aren't actually spicy, but they are packed with a fragrant spice blend that really gives these kebabs an authentic flare. (If you do want them spicy, simply add a bit of cayenne.) I just can't decide if I like the kebabs or the tangy yogurt sauce better. All I know is, they are absolutely harmonious together. Warm spices, juicy steak, smoky veggies and a creamy sauce—need I say more?

Try pairing this with the Lemony Spice-Roasted Mixed Veggies on page 130.

serves
3

active cooking time
30 minutes

total time
30 minutes

macros per serving

calories
518

protein
49.6 g

fat
30.8 g

net carbs
5.9 g

dill yogurt drizzle
½ cup (120 ml) plain Greek yogurt

1 tbsp (15 ml) fresh lemon juice (from ½ lemon)

1 tbsp (15 ml) water

¼ tsp sea salt

1 tsp dried dill

Note: For this recipe, you'll need four to five skewers. If you are using wooden skewers, add them to a drinking glass filled with water and let them soak for a couple of minutes on each end. This will prevent the skewers from burning.

spiced kebabs
1 tsp sea salt

½ tsp freshly cracked black pepper

2 tsp (4 g) sweet paprika

1 tsp garlic powder

⅛ tsp cinnamon

1½ lb (680 g) top sirloin steak, cut into 1" (2.5-cm) cubes (see Pro Tip)

1 bell pepper, cut into 1" (2.5-cm) squares

1 red onion, peeled and cut into 1" (2.5-cm) pieces

Nonstick cooking spray

To make the yogurt sauce, in a small bowl, add the yogurt, lemon juice, water, salt and dill. Stir until evenly mixed. Set it aside while you make the kebabs.

To make the kebabs, in a large bowl, add the salt, black pepper, paprika, garlic powder and cinnamon, and mix together. Add the cubes of beef and toss until they are evenly coated in the spices. Assemble the skewers by threading one piece of steak, one piece of pepper and one piece of onion onto the skewer. Repeat this pattern until you have four pieces of steak on each skewer.

Warm the grill (or indoor grill pan) over high heat. Once hot, grease the grates with nonstick cooking spray, and place the kebabs on the grill. Cook for 2 minutes, then rotate the skewer to the next side. If you're using an indoor grill pan, leave them on for 3 minutes on each side. Repeat the process until all four sides of the kebabs have cooked. Depending on the temperature of your grill and the thickness of your steak, this should take 8 to 10 minutes in total for medium-rare. If you're using an indoor grill pan, it will take 12 to 14 minutes. Take the skewers off the grill, and place them on a large plate or platter. Drizzle the kebabs with a little yogurt sauce, and serve with extra sauce on the side.

pro tip: For extra-tender kebabs, splurge on beef tenderloin or even lamb loin. You can also use chicken, but make sure to cook the skewers a bit longer for chicken to make sure they fully cook through to 165°F (75°C).

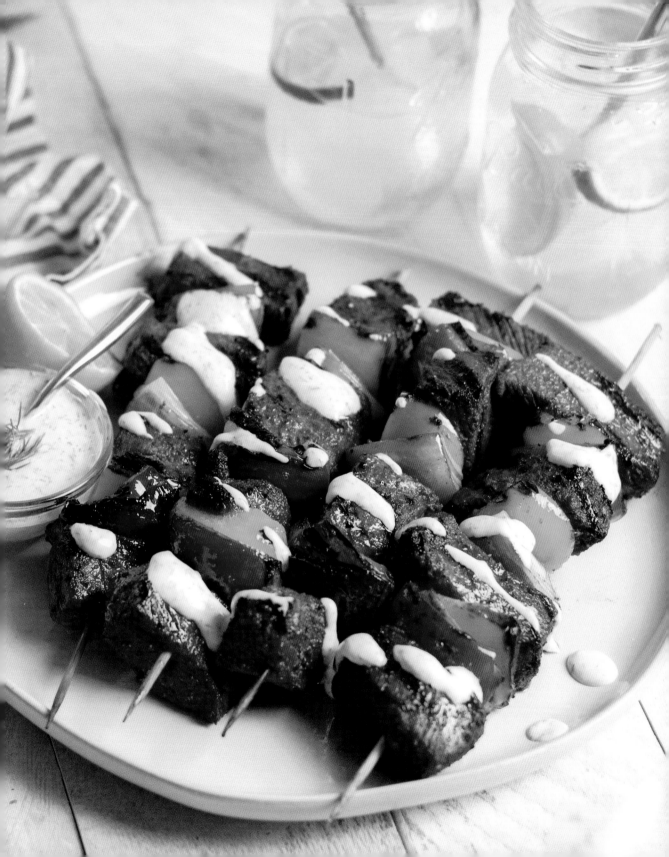

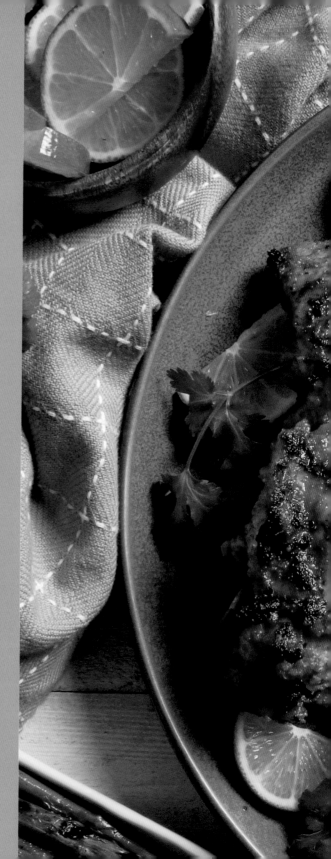

choice chicken

I know that for many, chicken can seem mundane. But not here—these are some cluckin' good recipes! This chapter is full of flavorful and exciting chicken dishes that will make your whole family smile. From garlicky wings to spicy firecracker meatballs, this menu has everyone covered.

Mike's Famous Bourbon Chicken (page 38)

Firecracker Chicken Meatballs (page 41)

The Perfect Garlic Parmesan Wings (page 42)

Piece-of-Cake Chicken Bake (page 45)

Zesty "Honey Mustard" Chicken (page 46)

Low-Carb Barbecue Chicken Tortilla Pizzas (page 49)

Quick Chicken Parm (page 50)

Thai Green Curry in a Hurry (page 53)

My Big Fat Greek Sheet-Pan Chicken (page 54)

Parmesan-Crusted Chicken Piccata (page 57)

Chili-Lime Grilled Chicken with Garlicky Aioli (page 58)

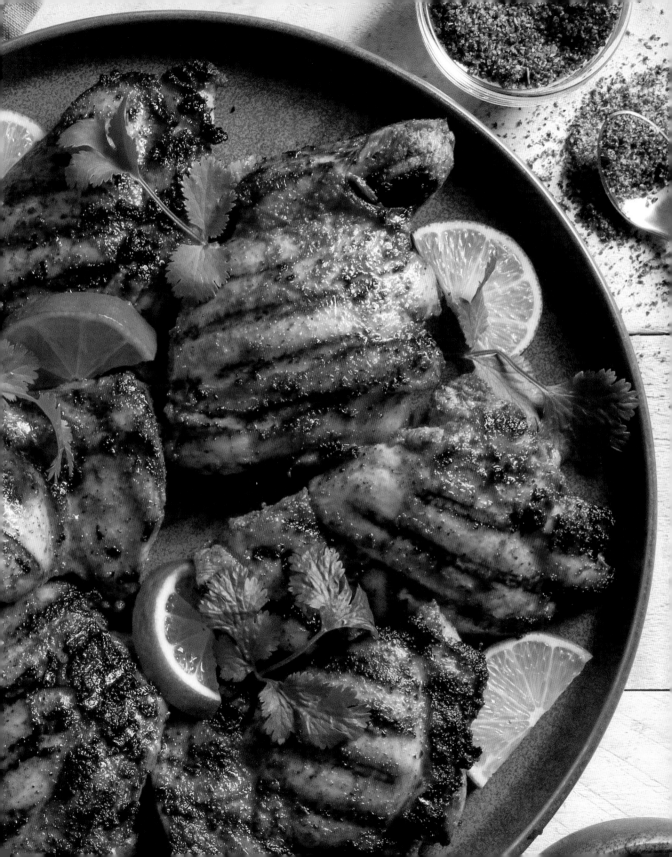

mike's famous bourbon chicken

As an angsty teenager (many, many years ago), nothing was "cooler" than endlessly wandering the corridors of the mall, and hitting up the food court was always essential. I made sure to get the free sample of bourbon chicken on a toothpick and inevitably ordered a big Styrofoam tray of it. Well, now you can have that nostalgic bite at home and this time without all the sugar! This recipe is now on weekly rotation at my house and I suspect it will be at yours too. It's easy, ridiculously tasty and really fun to make—Styrofoam optional. Fun Fact: The bourbon chicken name comes from Bourbon Street in New Orleans, not the liquor, so adding the bourbon in the recipe is totally optional.

Try pairing this with the Amazing Keto Pork Fried Rice on page 69.

¼ cup (60 ml) low-sodium soy sauce

¼ cup (54 g) granulated sweetener (I recommend allulose)

¼ cup (60 ml) sugar-free ketchup

2 tbsp (30 ml) water

2 tbsp (30 ml) bourbon (optional)

½ tsp sea salt

½ tsp freshly cracked black pepper

½ tsp ground ginger

2 tsp (4 g) sweet paprika

1½ tbsp (12 g) garlic powder

2 lb (907 g) boneless, skinless chicken thighs, diced into ½" (1-cm) cubes

2 tbsp (30 ml) avocado oil

1 scallion, thinly sliced, for garnish

In a large bowl, combine the soy sauce, sweetener, ketchup, water, bourbon (if using), salt, black pepper, ginger, paprika and garlic powder. Stir in the diced chicken until it's evenly coated in marinade and cover the bowl with plastic wrap. Set it in the fridge to marinate for a minimum of 5 minutes. Optionally, you can make this a day ahead and let it marinate overnight to get even more flavor.

Heat the avocado oil in a large (12-inch [30-cm]) nonstick pan over high heat. Once the oil is smoking hot, add the chicken, including all of the marinade. Spread the chicken in an even layer and let it sear for 5 minutes. Once the liquid has mostly evaporated, cook for 5 minutes, or until the chicken is nicely browned. You'll know it's done when the edges are turning a darker brown color and the liquid in the pan is completely gone. Turn off the heat and spoon the chicken into a serving bowl. Sprinkle the sliced scallions on top for garnish.

pro tip: If you prefer white meat chicken, you can cube boneless chicken tenders or breasts. Just shorten the overall cooking time by 1 to 2 minutes, as white meat cooks slightly faster than dark meat. You can also try this with salmon or shrimp!

serves
4

active cooking time
20 minutes

total time
25 minutes

macros per serving

calories
397

protein
50.9 g

fat
17.2 g

net carbs
2.7 g

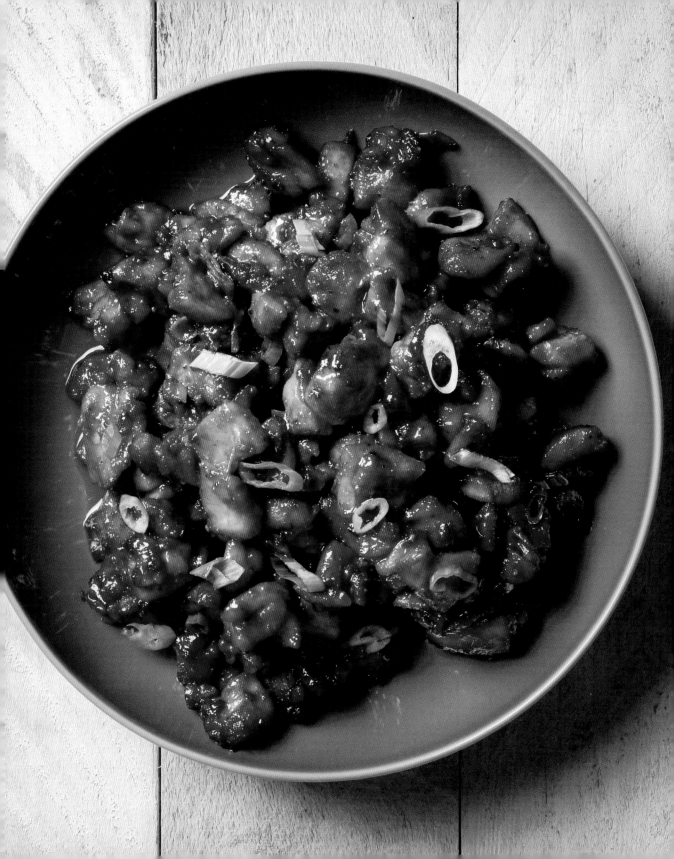

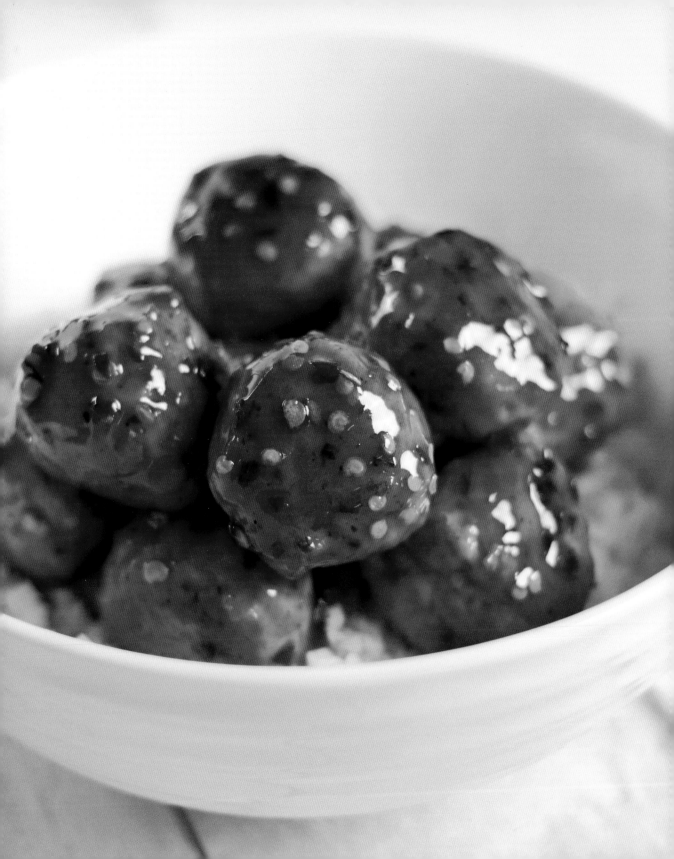

firecracker chicken meatballs

This recipe is for spice lovers like me. The flavors are simply addicting—sweet, spicy and tangy—it just hits every note. In fact, I'd suggest doubling the sauce and saving half for another day. It'll last up to 2 weeks in the fridge in an airtight jar. You can serve these meatballs over cauli-rice or with any veggies, but honestly, I just like eating them on their own right out of the pot. And if you don't have time to roll the meatballs yourself, check out the Pro Tip for an even speedier option.

Try pairing these with the Blistered Sichuan-Style Green Beans on page 122.

Try pairing these with the Blistered Sichuan-Style Green Beans on page 122.

serves
4

active cooking time
25 minutes

total time
25 minutes

macros per serving

calories
497

protein
46.6 g

fat
37 g

net carbs
2.2 g

chicken meatballs

1 lb (907 g) ground chicken (or turkey)

1 egg

2 tbsp (30 ml) mayonnaise

1 tsp sea salt

1 tsp freshly cracked black pepper

1 tbsp (8 g) garlic powder

1 tsp dried oregano

¼ cup (28 g) almond flour

2 tbsp (30 ml) avocado oil

firecracker sauce

½ cup (120 ml) Frank's RedHot sauce

2 tbsp (30 ml) apple cider vinegar

1 tbsp (14 g) unsalted butter (omit for dairy-free)

¼ tsp sea salt

1–2 tsp (2–4 g) crushed red pepper flakes (depending on desired spice level)

½ cup (72 g) packed brown sweetener (I recommend Swerve brand) or light brown sugar (110 g)

To make the meatballs, in large bowl, add the ground chicken, egg, mayonnaise, salt, black pepper, garlic powder, oregano and almond flour. Use your hands (I like to use rubber gloves for easy cleanup) to mix and massage everything together until evenly combined. Then, use the palms of your hands to roll the mixture into meatballs, no more than 1¼ inches (3 cm) in diameter, and set them aside on a pan or board. *Note: If the chicken mixture is too sticky to roll, add an extra tablespoon or two (7 or 14 g) of almond flour to the mixture and try again.*

Place a large nonstick pan over medium-high heat and add the avocado oil. Once hot, sear the meatballs in the pan for 5 to 6 minutes, or until the internal temperature of the meatballs reaches 165°F (75°C). Make sure to rotate them every minute or so until they're brown on all sides. You may need to cook the meatballs in two batches depending on the size of your pan. Once cooked through, set them aside on a plate to rest. Pour out any excess oil from the pan.

To make the firecracker sauce, place the same pan over medium heat and add the hot sauce, vinegar, butter, salt, red pepper flakes and brown sweetener. Whisk continuously for 1 minute, or until the sauce gets thick and bubbly. Turn off the heat and add the meatballs, tossing them around in the sauce until completely coated. Place the meatballs in a serving bowl and serve family-style.

pro tip: The firecracker sauce goes well with just about anything. Try it on wings, steak or even shrimp. If you're in a hurry and don't have time to make the meatballs, simply swap the ground chicken for chicken thighs or tenders. Dice them up into small cubes, toss with the same seasonings listed above and sauté them until cooked through. Then slather them in the sauce!

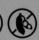

serves
4

active cooking
time
25 minutes

total time
30 minutes

macros per
serving

calories
604

protein
40.3 g

fat
50.5 g

net carbs
2.1 g

the perfect garlic parmesan wings

Maybe it's just me, but I think that the garlic Parmesan wings I order from the pizza sho are just never garlicky or Parmesan-y enough. So let's change that! These are the wing you've been dreaming of. Smothered in salty Parmesan and a heavy dose of garli these wings have all the crunch and juiciness of your favorite restaurant-style wings, b without the flour coating. The air fryer makes this quick and easy too, but you can bak them if you don't have one.

Try pairing this with the Loaded Lemon-Pepper Broccoli Salad on page 111.

chicken wings

2 lb (907 g) chicken wing drumettes and/or flats

1 tbsp (15 ml) avocado oil

1 tsp baking powder

2 tsp (12 g) seasoning salt or adobo

1 tsp garlic powder

Nonstick cooking spray

garlic parmesan sauce

¼ cup (60 ml) melted salted butter

4 cloves garlic, finely minced

½ tsp freshly cracked black pepper

¼ tsp crushed red pepper flakes

½ cup (50 g) grated Parmesan, plus extra for garnish

1 tbsp (4 g) finely chopped fresh Italian parsley

Preheat the air fryer to 400°F (200°C) or see the Pro Tip below if using an oven.

In a large bowl, add the wings, avocado oil, baking powder, seasoning salt and garlic powder. To the wings really well in the bowl to cover completely in the spices. Lightly spray the air fryer tray(s) wi cooking spray. Place the wings onto the tray(s) in an even layer. Make sure the wings have a little spac between them to allow the air to circulate—this will help the wings get nice and crispy. Cook them i the air fryer for 20 to 22 minutes, flipping them halfway through, or until they are golden brown an crispy.

While the wings cook, make the garlic Parmesan sauce by adding the melted butter, garlic, blac pepper, red pepper flakes, Parmesan and parsley to a large bowl. Whisk extremely well until complete combined. When all the wings are done, add them directly to the sauce and toss in the bowl unt they are fully coated. Pour the sauced wings onto a platter, garnish with extra Parmesan and serv family-style.

pro tip: If you don't have an air fryer, simply bake the wings in the oven at 350°F (180°C) for 25 minutes, flipping them halfway through. For a spicy kick, add 2 tablespoons (30 ml) of Frank's RedHot to the sauce mixture to make hot garlic Parm wings. For a creamier version, add 2 tablespoons (30 ml) of ranch or blue cheese dressing.

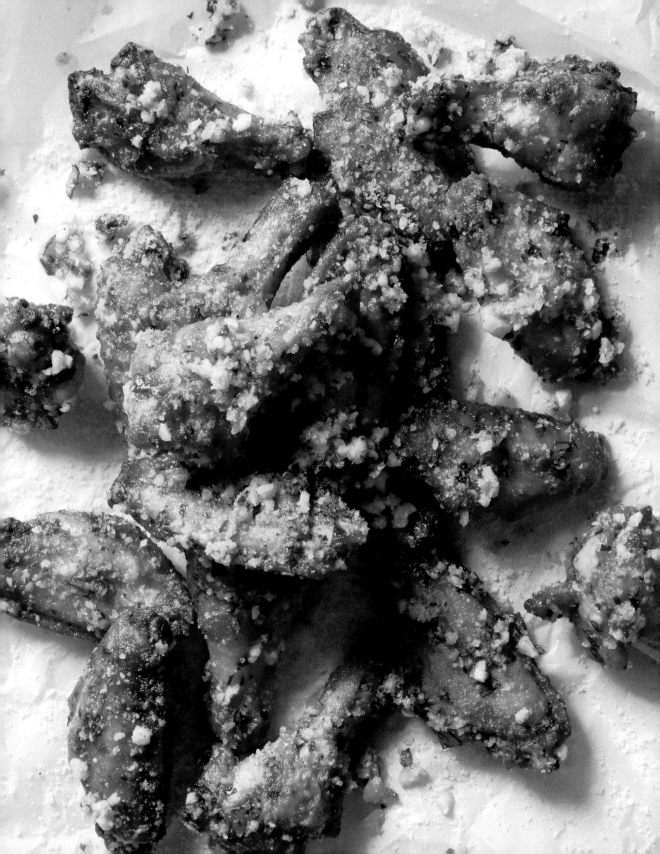

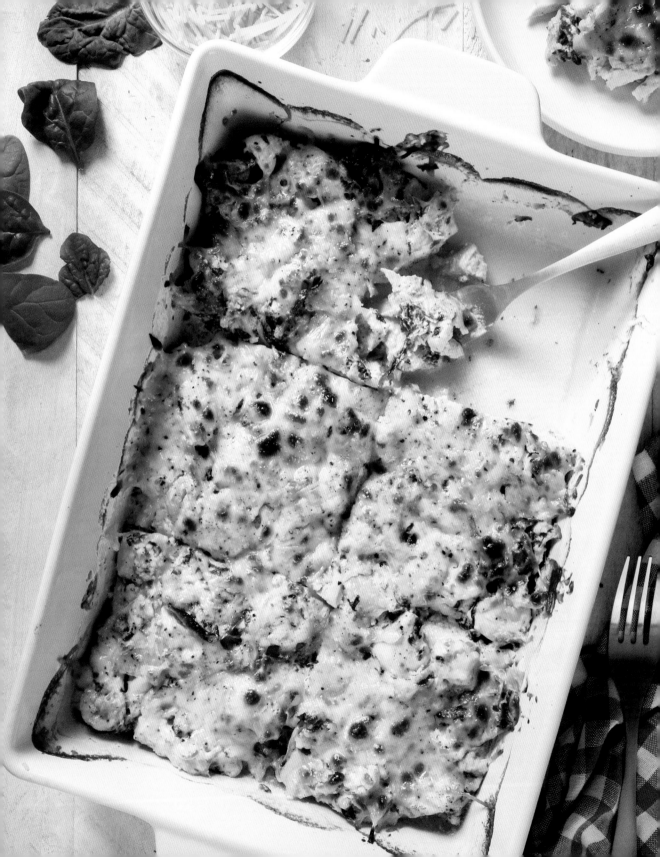

iece-of-cake chicken bake

ay, I'll admit it. Some nights, after a long day of working, even I don't feel like
king. We've all been there; you're definitely not alone. So, the next time you just
n't feel like making dinner, this is the recipe for you. This dish uses store-bought
nach dip as a serious shortcut to achieving something delicious without much effort.
mply mix the ingredients together, add them to a baking dish and walk away. A half-
ur later, a bubbly dinner will be waiting for you in the oven. It's as easy as pie . . . or
her . . . it's a piece of cake! And it's loaded with spinach for some extra nutrition and
vered in gooey cheese for some extra yumminess. So dig in and enjoy. It really doesn't
much easier than this.

pairing this with the **Herby Pan-Roasted Mushrooms** on page 126.

b (907 g) boneless, skinless chicken tenders
breasts

16-oz [454-g]) container spinach and
ichoke dip (see Pro Tip)

up (30 g) packed fresh baby spinach

tsp freshly cracked black pepper, divided

1 tsp garlic powder

¼ tsp crushed red pepper flakes (optional)

½ tsp dried oregano

½ cup (50 g) shredded or grated Parmesan
cheese, divided

1 cup (112 g) shredded mozzarella cheese

ke the chicken out of the fridge 15 minutes prior to cooking. Preheat the oven to 475°F (240°C) and
epare your oven rack to the upper position.

ut the chicken into 1-inch (2.5-cm) pieces, and place them in a large bowl with the dip, spinach,
teaspoon of the black pepper, garlic powder, red pepper flakes (if using), oregano and ¼ cup (25 g)
the Parmesan. Mix really well.

ur the chicken mixture into a 9 x 12–inch (23 x 30–cm) baking dish and spread it in one even layer.
p with the mozzarella and the remaining black pepper and Parmesan. Cover the dish with aluminum
l and place it on the upper rack of the oven. Bake for 20 minutes, and then remove the foil. Cook
5 minutes, or until the center of the dish is 165°F (75°C) using a meat thermometer, and the cheese
top is brown and bubbly throughout. Take the dish out of the oven and serve family-style while hot.

pro tip: This recipe is designed to be super quick and easy, but if you're feeling
"chefy" today, you can make your own spinach and artichoke dip from scratch by mixing
the following together in a bowl: 8 ounces (226 g) of cream cheese, ½ cup (120 ml) of
sour cream, ¼ cup (60 ml) of mayo, 1 (14-ounce [397-g]) can of quartered artichoke
hearts, 10 ounces (283 g) of frozen chopped spinach (thawed), 2 teaspoons (4 g) of
garlic powder and ¼ teaspoon each of salt and pepper.

serves
6

**active cooking
time**
25 minutes

total time
35 minutes

**macros per
serving**

calories
435

protein
46 g

fat
19.5 g

net carbs
4.8 g

serves
4

active cooking time
25 minutes

total time
25 minutes

macros per serving

calories
606

protein
71.6 g

fat
30.8 g

net carbs
2.2 g

zesty "honey mustard" chicken

There is just something special about this recipe. It takes humble chicken breast and turns it into something memorable. The sauce is so bright and tangy, and the beautiful golden color is just so inviting. To avoid the added sugars, there is no honey mustard in this recipe . . . but you'd never know it, because it tastes exactly like a real honey mustard dressing. In fact, it's even better! This simple recipe is super easy to make but tastes complex and sophisticated. And because it's sugar-free, you can really soak up all that yummy sauce!

Try pairing this with the Sweet Balsamic-Glazed Brussels on page 121.

2½ lb (1.1 kg) boneless chicken breasts
(4 pieces; see Pro Tip)

1 tsp sea salt

½ tsp freshly cracked black pepper

2 tbsp (30 ml) avocado oil

1 cup (240 ml) heavy cream or coconut cream
(for dairy-free)

¼ cup (60 ml) Dijon mustard

3 tbsp (45 ml) whole-grain mustard (I recommend
Maille Old Style mustard)

½ cup (108 g) granulated sweetener
(I recommend allulose)

Take the chicken out of the fridge about 15 minutes ahead to temper. Warm a large (12-inch [30-cm] cast-iron skillet or nonstick pan over medium-high heat. While the pan warms up, season the chicken evenly on all sides with the salt and black pepper. Once the pan is smoking hot, add the avocado oil and the chicken. Sear the chicken for 5 minutes on each side, or until both sides have a nice golden brown crust. Remove the chicken from the pan and set it aside on a plate. *Note: The chicken may not be fully cooked at this point, so please don't eat it yet!*

Pour out and discard any grease left in the pan, and then place it back on the stove over medium-low heat. Add the heavy cream, Dijon mustard, whole-grain mustard and sweetener, and whisk until everything is fully combined. Bring the sauce to a gentle simmer, and then place the chicken back in the pan. Turn the heat down to low and let the chicken simmer with the sauce for 5 minutes, flipping halfway through. For perfectly cooked chicken, look for an internal temperature of 165°F (75°C), using a meat thermometer. Remove the pan from the heat and spoon some extra sauce over the top of the chicken before serving family-style from the pan or in a nice serving dish.

pro tip: Instead of chicken, try this recipe with salmon. The salmon is absolutely wonderful in the "honey mustard" sauce. Simply sear skinless salmon fillets for 5 to 6 minutes on each side before adding them into the zesty sauce.

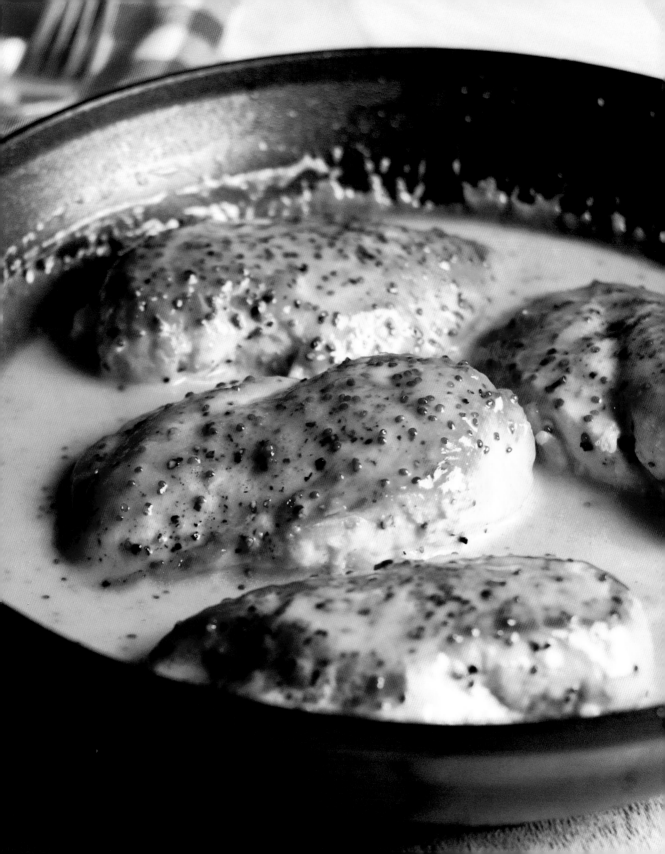

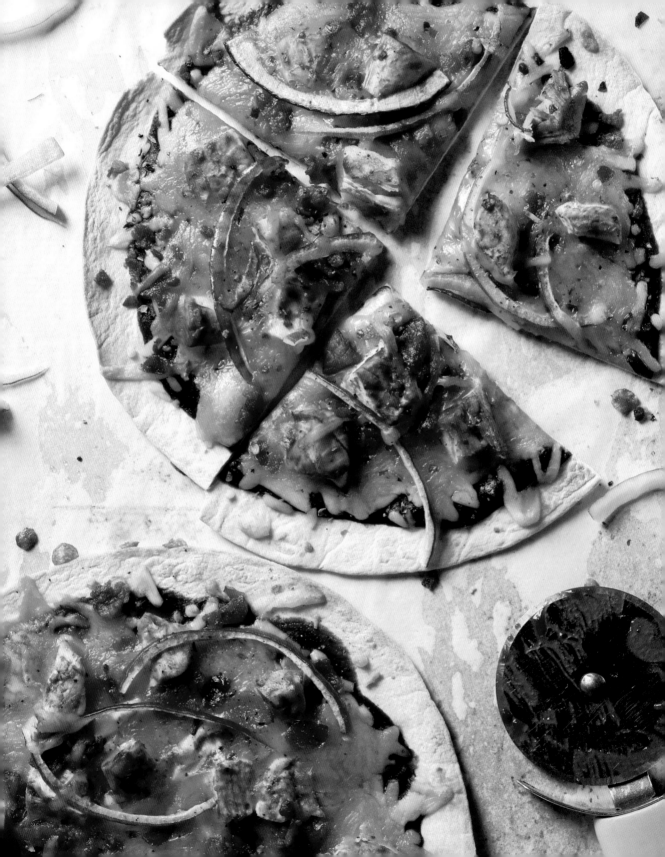

low-carb barbecue chicken tortilla pizzas

This family-friendly recipe is so quick and easy, even the kids will want to jump in and help! It's fun and customizable, so everyone can top these personal-sized pizzas however they want. And don't be surprised when the family asks for these over and over again. They are simply delicious and much healthier (and more budget friendly) than your typical pizza options. So, the next time it's pizza night, skip the delivery and try this recipe instead!

4 (8" [20-cm]) low-carb tortillas (see Pro Tips)

1½ cups (355 g) cooked rotisserie chicken meat (see Pro Tips)

½ cup (120 ml) no-sugar barbecue sauce, divided (I recommend Sweet Baby Ray's brand)

2 cups (224 g) shredded Colby and Monterey Jack cheese blend or Cheddar

¼ red onion, thinly sliced

¼ cup (28 g) bacon pieces/bits

¼ tsp freshly cracked black pepper

¼ tsp dried oregano

¼ tsp crushed red pepper flakes

Preheat the oven to 400°F (200°C). Line two baking sheets with parchment paper or aluminum foil.

Place the tortillas onto the baking sheets and set aside. Dice the chicken into ½-inch (1.3-cm) cubes. Place the chicken in a bowl, and toss it with 2 tablespoons (30 ml) of the barbecue sauce, until evenly coated. Spread the remaining barbecue sauce, divided four ways, onto the tortillas. I like to leave a small, empty border around the edges of the tortillas, almost like the typical pizza crust. Top the pizzas evenly with the chicken, cheese, onion, bacon, black pepper, oregano and red pepper flakes. Place the sheets into the oven and bake for 7 minutes, or until the cheese is fully melted. Remove the tray from the oven and cut each pizza into four slices before serving.

pro tips: For a crispier crust, prebake the tortillas first by placing them on a baking sheet and tossing them in the oven for 5 minutes before adding all the toppings.

If you want to use fresh chicken instead of store-bought, season 1 pound (454 g) of boneless chicken tenders with ¼ teaspoon of salt and pepper, and sear them in a pan over medium-high heat for 5 minutes, or just until cooked through. Then slice them into bite-sized pieces before adding them along with the pizza toppings.

serves
4

active cooking time
20 minutes

total time
30 minutes

macros per serving

calories
530

protein
64.3 g

fat
26.2 g

net carbs
6.8 g

quick chicken parm

My dad is like my best friend. He's not only our family's "professional advisor" (he really does give the best advice), but he's also our resident comedian. My entire life he's taught me the importance of a good laugh, even in the toughest of times. It's something I tremendously admire about him. He's basically taught me everything I know, but most critically, he's taught me that there really isn't anything better than a perfect chicken parm! Dad, this recipe is for you. I've taken your favorite food in the world and given it my own spin, with a healthy twist, of course. It's not breaded, nor is it served on a mountain of pasta, but it is equally as delicious. And it's quick enough to make any night of the week.

Try pairing this with The Ultimate Blackened Chicken Caesar Salad on page 107.

2 lb (907 g) thin-sliced boneless chicken breasts (see Pro Tip)

1 tsp sea salt

½ tsp freshly cracked black pepper

1 tsp garlic powder

½ tsp dried Italian herb blend or oregano

2 tbsp (30 ml) avocado oil

1 (24-oz [680-g]) jar no-sugar marinara (I recommend Rao's brand)

8 oz (226 g) fresh mozzarella, pre-sliced or sliced thinly

2 tbsp (13 g) grated Parmesan

Thinly-sliced basil, to serve (optional)

Take the chicken out of the fridge 15 minutes ahead to temper. Preheat the oven to 425°F (215°C).

Place a large (12-inch [30-cm]) skillet over medium-high heat. While the skillet warms up, season both sides of the chicken with the salt, black pepper, garlic powder and Italian herb blend. Once the pan is smoking hot, add the avocado oil and carefully place the chicken in the pan. Sear the chicken for 3 to 4 minutes on each side, or until the chicken gets a golden brown crust. When the chicken is cooked, set it aside on a plate to rest.

In a 9 x 13–inch (23 x 33–cm) baking dish, pour in the marinara sauce, spreading it in an even layer. Nestle the chicken breasts into the sauce and top each breast with the sliced mozzarella. Place the baking dish in the oven, uncovered, and bake for 12 minutes, or just until the sauce is bubbly on the edges and the cheese is melted. Take the chicken out of the oven, sprinkle it with the Parmesan cheese and fresh basil (if using), and serve it family-style.

pro tip: If you can't find thin-sliced chicken breasts, simply butterfly or slice whole chicken breasts in half, horizontally. You can also pound out boneless chicken breasts or tenders until they're about ½ inch (1.3 cm) thick. This helps tenderize the meat and keep it extra juicy.

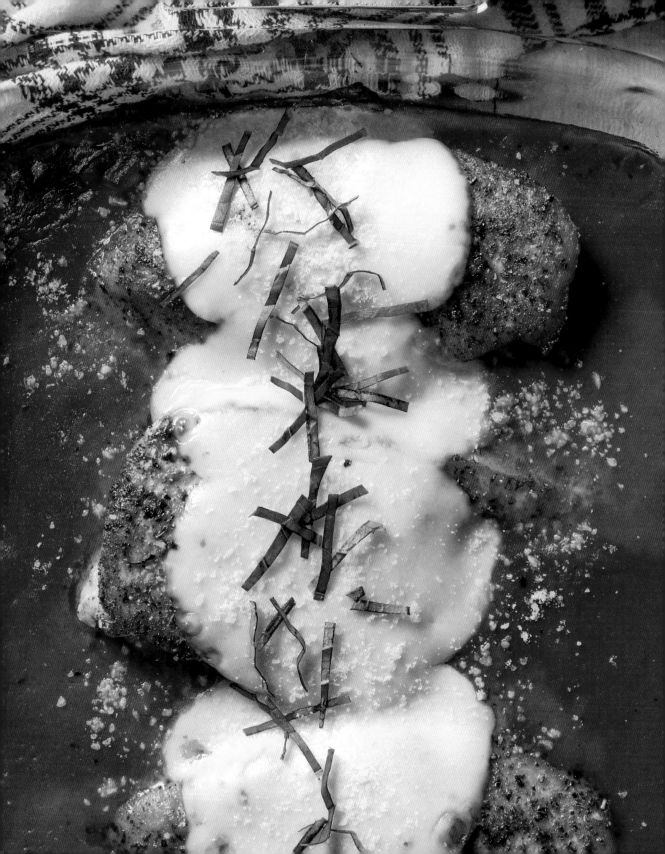

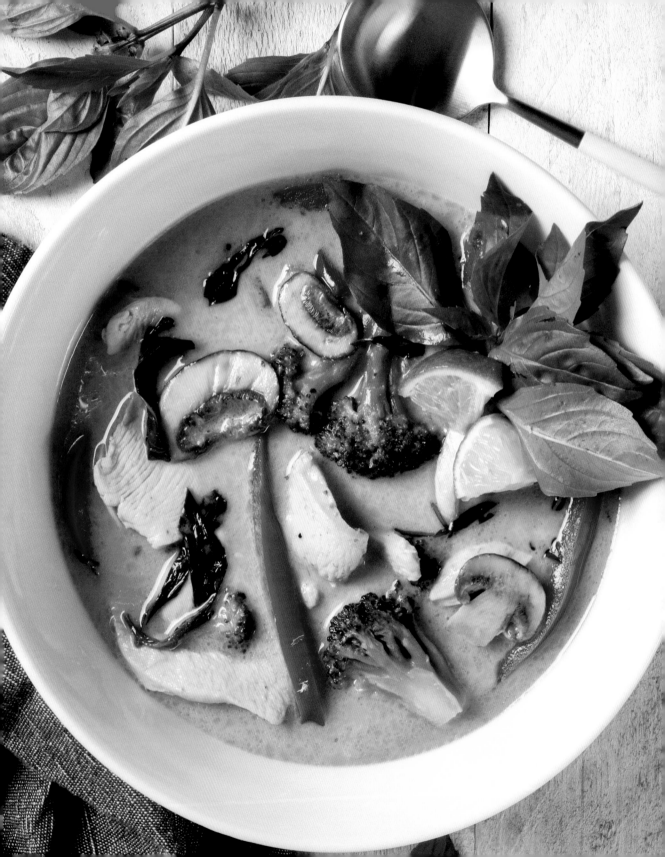

thai green curry in a hurry

Thai food can seem challenging to make at home, especially considering how beautifully bold the dishes are. But this recipe will show you that you can absolutely do it! In fact, it's surprisingly approachable. In Thailand, I learned how to make green curry paste from scratch, and hey, if you're up for it, I won't stop you! But I call this "curry in a hurry" for a reason: It's designed to be quick! So yes, I skip a few steps normally used in an authentic green curry, but the flavors still pack a huge punch. And even without the sugar, this dinner leaves nothing to be desired. Creamy, spicy and herbaceous, this bowl of heaven is sure to put a smile on your face. After all, there's a reason Thailand is known as "the land of smiles."

2 tbsp (30 ml) melted coconut oil or avocado oil

3–4 tbsp (45–60 g) green curry paste (I recommend Maesri brand)

1 (13.5-oz [398 ml]) can unsweetened coconut milk

2 tbsp (30 ml) fresh lime juice (from 2 limes)

2 tbsp (30 ml) fish sauce

1 lb (454 g) boneless chicken breasts, thinly sliced

1 red bell pepper, thinly sliced

1 cup (70 g) pre-sliced cremini mushrooms

1 cup (91 g) frozen broccoli florets

¼ cup (6 g) packed Thai basil with stems removed, plus extra for garnish

In a saucepan over medium heat, add the coconut oil. Once hot, add the curry paste and use a spoon or spatula to break apart and fry the paste for 2 minutes, or until it starts to just slightly brown. Immediately pour in the coconut milk, stirring well to combine the sauce. Add the lime juice and fish sauce, and bring to a gentle boil. Stir in the chicken, bring everything back to a gentle boil and simmer for 3 minutes. Stir in the bell pepper and mushrooms and boil for 2 minutes. Stir in the broccoli and basil, and simmer for 2 minutes, or until the broccoli is fully cooked. To serve, pour the curry into bowls and garnish with lime wedges and/or more Thai basil.

pro tip: For extra yumminess, you can add any of the following optional ingredients: whole baby corn, green beans, sliced eggplant, tofu, sliced grape tomatoes and/or sliced red or green jalapeños (for those who really like it spicy!). Simply stir them in along with the bell peppers and mushrooms in this recipe.

serves
2

active cooking time
25 minutes

total time
25 minutes

macros per serving

calories
435

protein
55.4 g

fat
20.1 g

net carbs
8.5 g

my big fat greek sheet-pan chicken

Tired of the same ol', same ol' chicken dinner? Well this is the recipe for you. Sure, th[is] dish is quick and easy—after all, you just toss everything on a sheet tray and pop it [in] the oven—but it's so much more than that. This is a flavor-packed party-on-a-plate. (Sa[y] that three times fast.) The briny olives, punchy pepperoncini and salty Feta join force[s] to make this one exciting meal. And no need for sides here, because this sheet-tray h[as] everything you need to feed your family quickly and deliciously!

serves
4

active cooking time
10 minutes

total time
30 minutes

macros per serving

calories
495

protein
40.7 g

fat
30.1 g

net carbs
7.9 g

¼ cup (60 ml) extra virgin olive oil

¼ cup (60 ml) fresh lemon juice (from 2 lemons)

1 tsp sea salt

½ tsp freshly cracked black pepper

1 tbsp (8 g) garlic powder

1½ tbsp (8 g) dried oregano

2 lb (907 g) boneless, skinless chicken thighs

1 cup (149 g) grape tomatoes

½ red onion, sliced

8 oz (226 g) pepperoncini, drained

½ cup (90 g) drained pitted Kalamata or green olives

¼ cup (38 g) crumbled Feta cheese (optional)

Preheat the oven to 450°F (230°C) and line a baking sheet with parchment paper or aluminum foil.

In a large bowl, add the olive oil, lemon juice, salt, black pepper, garlic powder and oregano, an[d] mix together well. Add the chicken and toss everything together until the chicken is evenly coated [in] the marinade, inside and out. Add the tomatoes, onion, pepperoncini and olives, and toss to ensu[re] everything is coated. Using tongs, place the chicken thighs onto the lined baking sheet with the to[p] sides up. Then, pour all the vegetable mixture into the open spaces around the chicken, spreadin[g] everything in an even layer. Make sure to drizzle any leftover marinade from the bowl on top of th[e] chicken and veggies.

Place the tray into the oven on the upper rack, and bake for 20 minutes, or until the internal temperatu[re] of the chicken is 165°F (75°C). Switch the oven to broil, and broil for 2 minutes, or until the top of th[e] chicken has a golden brown crust. Take the tray out of the oven, sprinkle the Feta cheese (if using) [all] over while it's still warm, and serve family-style.

pro tip: For a quick and easy version for two, simply halve this recipe and cook it in an air fryer at 400°F (200°C) for 20 minutes.

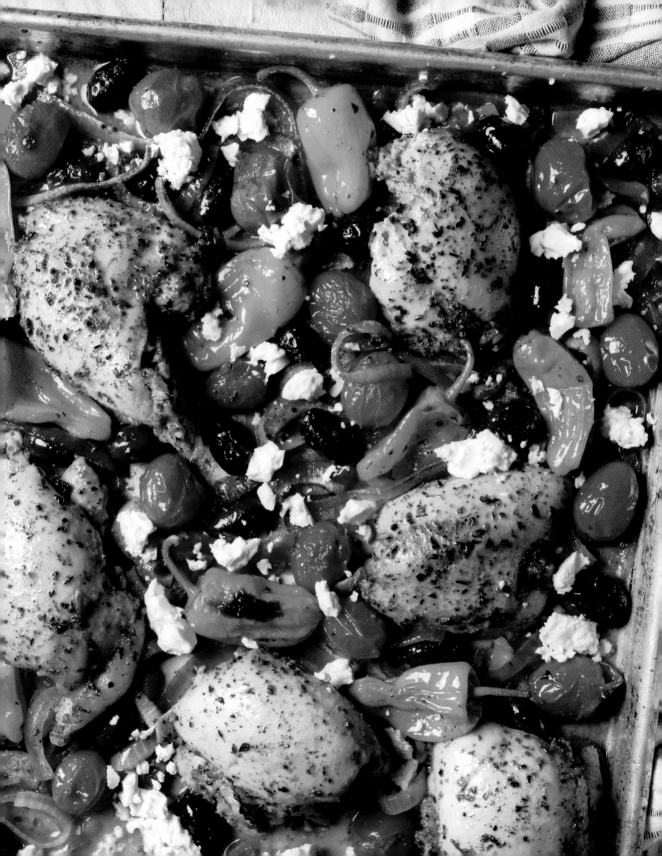

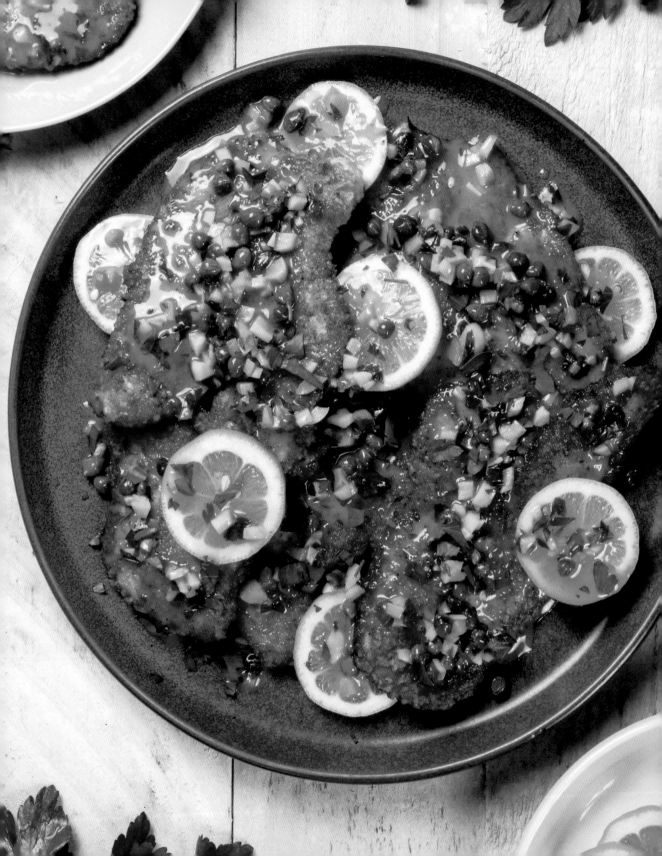

parmesan-crusted chicken piccata

We all have the one dish we crave when we're back "home." For me, that's my mom's chicken piccata. This was a staple in our house growing up, and I still think my mom's version is the best (obviously), but this is a close second! And instead of crusting the chicken in flour or breadcrumbs, this recipe uses grated Parmesan. It may seem like a small change, but it yields big results . . . without the carbs! The crust is flavorful and crispy, and it keeps the chicken juicy and delicious. The white wine lemon sauce is packed with zesty flavor, and the capers give it that perfect, salty finish with each bite. This is a taste of home, so I hope you love it as much as I do.

Try pairing this with the Beautifully Layered Eggplant Caprese on page 129.

Try pairing this with the Beautifully Layered Eggplant Caprese on page 129.

lb (907 g) thin-sliced boneless chicken breasts (see Pro Tip)

eggs, beaten

cup (100 g) grated Parmesan

tsp freshly cracked black pepper

tbsp (16 g) garlic powder

tbsp (15 ml) avocado oil

cup (120 ml) dry white wine

tbsp (15 ml) fresh lemon juice (from ½ lemon)

½ tsp chicken bouillon powder (I recommend Knorr® brand)

4 cloves garlic, chopped

3 tbsp (42 g) unsalted butter

2 tbsp (16 g) drained capers

¼ cup (15 g) packed chopped fresh Italian parsley

Sliced lemon, for garnish (optional)

Take the chicken out of the fridge 15 minutes ahead to temper. Set up your dredging station by beating the eggs in one bowl and mixing together the Parmesan, black pepper and garlic powder in a separate bowl. Dip each piece of chicken into the egg, shaking off any excess, and then press it into the Parmesan mixture and coat it on all sides. Once fully coated, set each piece of chicken aside on a plate.

Warm the avocado oil in a nonstick skillet over medium heat. When the oil is hot, swirl it around the pan to coat the bottom, and add the chicken. Don't overcrowd the pan—cook the chicken in two batches, if needed. Fry the chicken for 3 to 4 minutes on each side, or until the crust is browned and crispy. Don't move it around too much in the pan, as this will help ensure the "breading" sticks to the chicken. Once cooked, take the chicken out of the pan and set it aside on a large serving plate.

Discard the oil from the pan, and place the same pan over high heat. Meanwhile, mix together the white wine, lemon juice, chicken bouillon and garlic in a small bowl. When the pan is hot, pour the mixture into the pan and cook for 1 minute, stirring with a spoon. Add the butter and capers, and gently stir everything continuously until the butter is fully melted into the sauce. The sauce should become translucent white and thicken slightly. Turn off the heat and stir in the parsley. Just before serving, pour that delicious sauce all over the chicken. Garnish with slices of lemon (if using) and enjoy!

pro tip: If you can't find thin-sliced chicken breasts, simply butterfly or slice whole chicken breasts in half, horizontally. You can also pound out boneless chicken breasts or tenders until they're about ½ inch (1.3 cm) thick.

macros per serving

calories
540

protein
62.4 g

fat
26.2 g

net carbs
5.0 g

serves
4

active cooking time
25 minutes

total time
25 minutes

macros per serving

calories
510

protein
38.9 g

fat
35.1 g

net carbs
2.8 g

chili-lime grilled chicken with garlicky aioli

This dish is fun, festive and packed with juicy flavor. It's quick and easy too, so it work well for any weeknight dinner, but it's got a few flavorful twists that make this dis impressive enough for a dinner party or even your next grill-out. Serve with veggies an tortillas for some seriously awesome chicken tacos too. Don't have a grill? No problem Sear the chicken thighs on both sides in a skillet for 5 minutes on each side, or place them on a baking sheet and roast them in the oven at 450°F (230°C) for 20 minutes instead.

Try pairing this with the Fab 5-Minute Spanish Rice on page 125.

chili-lime chicken

2 lb (907 g) boneless, skinless chicken thighs

2 tbsp (30 ml) fresh lime juice (from 2 limes)

2 tbsp (30 ml) avocado oil

1 tsp sea salt

½ tsp freshly cracked black pepper

1 tbsp (8 g) garlic powder

1 tbsp (6 g) chili-lime seasoning (I recommend Tajín® brand)

2 tsp (4 g) chipotle powder (for spicy) or smoked paprika (for mild)

Nonstick cooking spray

garlicky cilantro lime aioli

½ cup (120 ml) mayonnaise

2 tbsp (30 ml) fresh lime juice (from 2 limes)

1 clove garlic, grated

2 tbsp (2 g) packed finely chopped fresh cilantro plus extra to serve (see Pro Tip)

Lime wedges, to serve (optional)

To marinate the chicken, add the chicken, lime juice, avocado oil, salt, black pepper, garlic powde chili-lime seasoning and chipotle powder to a gallon-sized freezer bag. Close the bag, removing th air, and use your hands to mix and massage the marinade into the meat. Set the bag aside to marinate for a minimum of 5 minutes, but you can make this a day ahead and let it marinate in the fridge overnight to get even more flavor.

To make the aioli, in a small bowl, add the mayonnaise, lime juice, garlic and cilantro. Mix well and set in the fridge to rest.

Warm an outdoor grill or indoor grill pan over high heat. Once it's smoking hot, lightly oil the grates c pan with the cooking spray. Place the chicken on the grill and cook for 4 to 5 minutes on each side or until the internal temperature of the chicken reaches 165°F (75°C). Once the chicken is done, set aside on a plate to rest before serving. Serve with the aioli on the side and garnish with lime wedge and cilantro (if using).

pro tip: Whenever you use fresh cilantro, don't be afraid to include the stems, because that's where ALL the flavor is! Simply chop them up along with the leaves. Note: This is not the case with most other fresh herbs such as parsley, rosemary and thyme. Aside from cilantro, removing the stems is recommended for most other fresh herbs.

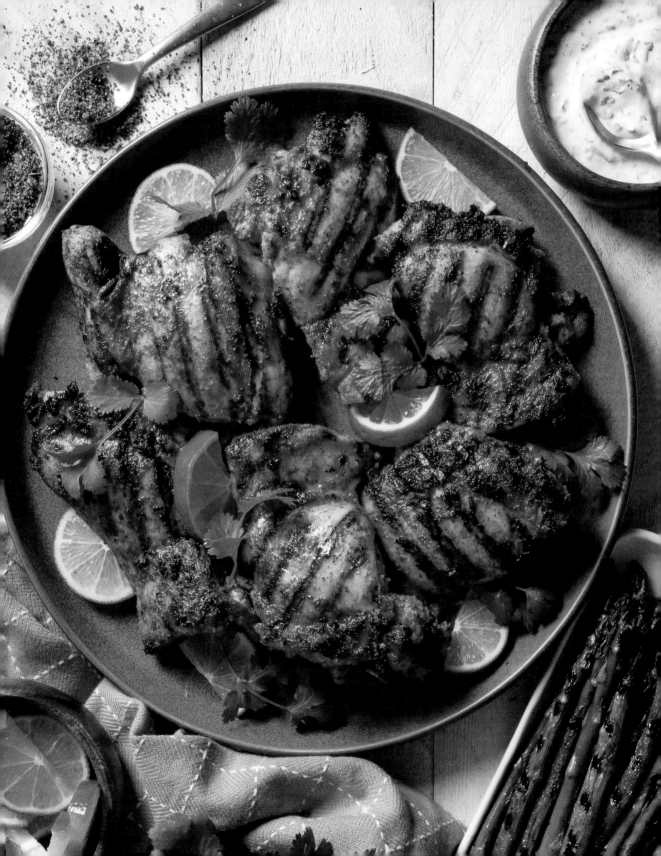

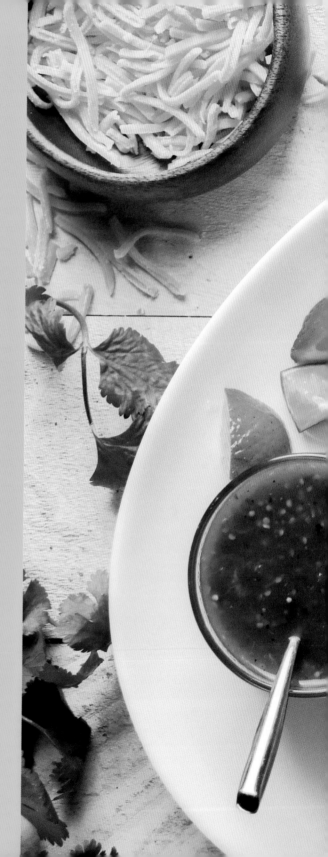

pronto pork

Sadly, pork is too often overlooked. Its big sisters, chicken and beef, seem to get all the limelight around here. And as the youngest of three siblings, I get it. But it's time for the humble pork to shine! And these recipes do just that. From tacos to fried rice, these pork dinners are here to show that pork is finger-lickin' good too!

Popcorn Pork Belly with Yum Yum Sauce (page 62)

Austin Food Truck Breakfast Tacos (for Dinner!) (page 65)

Spicy Italian Stuffed Banana Peppers (page 66)

Amazing Keto Pork Fried Rice (page 69)

Last-Minute Low-Carb "Al Pastor" Bowls (page 70)

Vibrant Thai-Style Pork Larb (page 73)

Pork Chops in Wicked Mardi Gras Sauce (page 74)

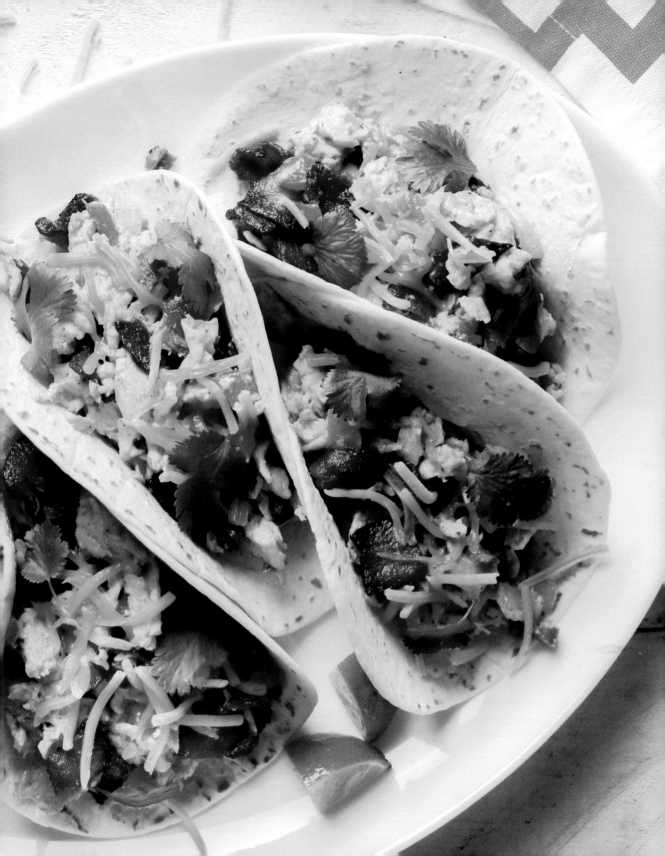

popcorn pork belly with yum yum sauce

Crunchy, juicy and super fun to eat, this kid- and adult-friendly recipe is just as good a it sounds—and it's a great alternative to breaded nuggets! The pork belly gives thes crispy bites an extra-rich and tender twist on a classic. And if you don't eat pork, this i still fantastic with chicken, shrimp or even salmon. Oh, and did I mention that the yur yum sauce is finger-lickin' good? Make a double batch and store the leftovers in a jar fo later. It will last up to 10 days in your fridge.

Try pairing this with the Blistered Sichuan-Style Green Beans on page 122.

serves
2

active cooking time
20 minutes

total time
25 minutes

macros per serving

calories
926

protein
13.3 g

fat
88.3 g

net carbs
2 g

popcorn pork belly
2 cups (60 g) unflavored pork rinds/chicharron
½ tsp freshly cracked black pepper
2 eggs
½ lb (226 g) skinless pork belly
Avocado oil for frying (optional)

yum yum sauce
¼ cup (60 ml) mayonnaise
1 tsp tomato paste

1 tsp low-sodium soy sauce
½ tsp Worcestershire sauce
1 tsp apple cider vinegar
1 tsp granulated sweetener (I recommend allulose)
1 tsp garlic powder
¼ tsp sweet paprika
¼ tsp ground ginger
½ tsp sriracha sauce (optional)

To make the pork belly, place the pork rinds in a plastic quart-sized freezer bag and tightly seal removing the air. Use a rolling pin or the back of a pan to gently beat the rinds until they turn into c breadcrumb-like powder (see Pro Tips). Pour the crumbs into a large bowl, stir in the black pepper and set the bowl aside. In another small bowl, whisk together the eggs and set that aside as well.

Slice the pork into ¾-inch (2-cm) cubes (see Pro Tips), and add them to the bowl with the eggs. Sti with a fork until the cubes are completely coated in the egg wash. Take three or four pieces at a time out of the egg wash, letting the excess drip off, and toss them in the crumbs until they are fully coated Set them aside on a plate, and repeat until all the pork belly cubes are covered and ready to cook.

Set the air fryer to 350°F (180°C) and place the pork onto the removable tray. Cook for 12 to 14 minutes or until the pork bites are golden brown, flipping them over halfway through. Don't have an air fryer? Par fry them in avocado oil for 3 minutes on each side, or until they are golden brown and crispy.

While the pork is cooking, make the sauce by combining in a small bowl the mayo, tomato paste, soy sauce, Worcestershire, vinegar, sweetener, garlic powder, paprika, ginger and sriracha (if using). Whisk well until the sauce is smooth and creamy. Take the finished popcorn pork out of the air frye and put it on a serving plate with the yum yum sauce on the side.

pro tips: To make this recipe even quicker, skip making your own "pork crumbs." Many grocery stores now sell them—look for Pork King Good® or Bacon's Heir® brands.

To make it easier to cut the pork belly, freeze it for about 15 minutes before you slice.

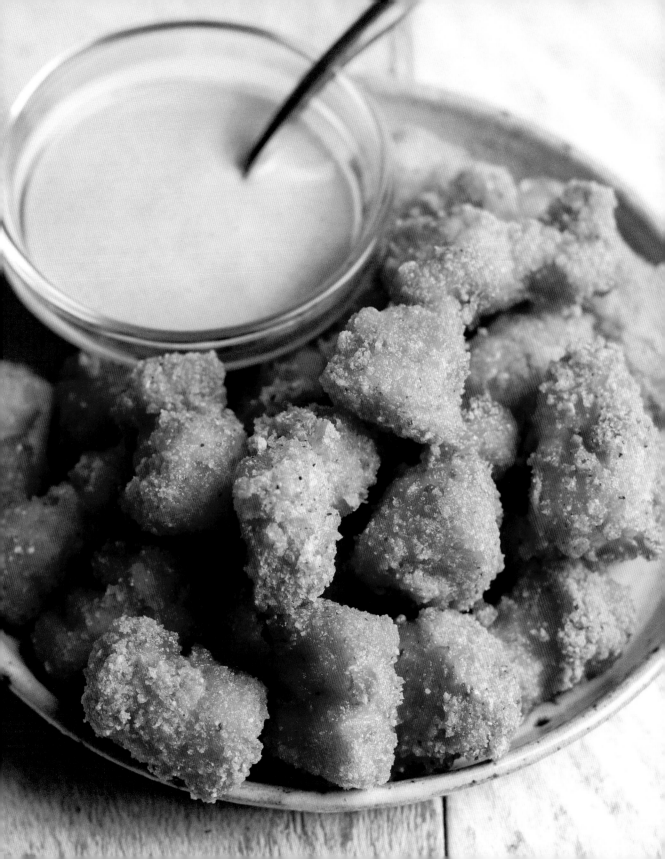

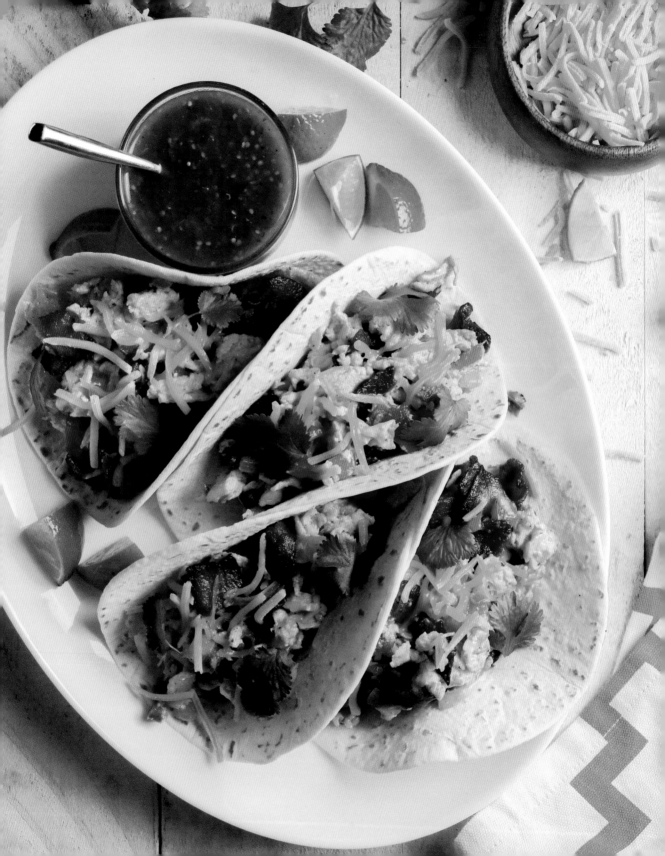

...ustin food truck breakfast tacos (...for dinner!)

...here is much debate here in Texas about who has the best breakfast tacos: Austin or San ...ntonio. And although I'm biased, Austin wins this battle. Here in Austin, if you aren't ...etting your breakfast tacos from a food truck, you just aren't doing it right. But for ...veryone else outside of Texas, this is the recipe for you. A good breakfast taco should ...e warm and wrapped in aluminum foil with the tortilla softly hugging the eggs, bacon ...nd cheese. It's simply the best. So naturally, I had to make my own version, with a few ...ealthier twists, to bring a taste of Austin to your kitchen. And don't let the name fool ...ou. These are not just for breakfast. They are the perfect, protein-packed meal for any ...me of day.

serves
3

active cooking time
25 minutes

total time
25 minutes

macros per serving

calories
557

protein
31.3 g

fat
29 g

net carbs
4.9 g

... (12-oz [340-g]) package no-sugar bacon
...ee Pro Tip)

... tbsp (30 ml) cold water

... eggs

... tsp sea salt, divided

... green or red bell pepper, diced

...-2 jalapeños, seeded and minced

... yellow onion, diced

1 clove garlic, minced

¼ tsp freshly cracked black pepper

6 small (taco-size) low-carb tortillas

½ cup (57 g) shredded Cheddar or pepper Jack cheese (optional)

Salsa verde, sour cream, hot sauce, cilantro, avocado and/or lime wedges, to serve (optional)

...ut the bacon into ½-inch (1.3-cm) pieces. Add the bacon pieces directly to a cold, nonstick pan ...0-inch [25-cm]), along with the water. Place the cold pan over medium heat. Let the bacon slowly ...ook for 8 minutes, stirring occasionally to separate the bacon pieces, or until the bacon is cooked to ...our liking. (I like mine extra crispy!) While the bacon is cooking, use this time to prep all your veggies, ...nd beat the eggs in a bowl with ½ teaspoon of the salt. Use a slotted spoon to remove the bacon ...om the pan and set it aside on a plate. Leave the bacon grease in the pan.

...ace the same pan back over medium heat, and add the bell pepper, jalapeños, onion, garlic, black ...epper and remaining salt. Sauté the veggies for 4 minutes, or just until the onion is translucent. (You ...vant to leave some "bite" to the veggies, which adds nice texture to the tacos.) Pour the eggs right into ...e pan on top of the veggies, and scramble the eggs for 1 minute, or until they're just cooked through. ...ull the pan off the heat and stir in the bacon.

...Varm the tortillas by lightly toasting them in a dry pan over medium-high heat for 10 seconds on each ...de, and set them onto a plate. To serve, add the taco filling to the tortillas, then top with the Cheddar ...heese (if using). Serve with your favorite fixin's. I like mine with cilantro and salsa verde.

pro tip: This recipe is also great if you have some leftover meat from dinner the night before. Swap the bacon for leftover steak, chicken or sausage, and it's taco time!

spicy italian stuffed banana peppers

serves
3

active cooking time
15 minutes

total time
45 minutes

macros per serving

calories
558

protein
37.2 g

fat
41 g

net carbs
6.7 g

Big, bold and spicy . . . these ain't your mama's stuffed peppers! These Italian sausage stuffed peppers are bursting with flavor and covered in gooey cheese. And they are fun and easy to make! The yellow peppers are vibrant and flavorful and look beautiful when they're cooked. And unlike typical stuffed peppers, these aren't laced with carb fillers like rice or breadcrumbs.

Try pairing this with the Beautifully Layered Eggplant Caprese on page 129.

6 Hungarian wax or banana peppers (about 1 lb [454 g]; see Pro Tip)

1 lb (454 g) mild or spicy ground Italian sausage

¼ tsp sea salt

¼ tsp freshly cracked black pepper

½ tsp crushed red pepper flakes

½ tsp dried oregano

1 tsp garlic powder

½ cup (56 g) shredded mozzarella cheese, divided

1 cup (240 ml) no-sugar marinara or pasta sauce (I recommend Rao's brand)

Preheat the oven to 475°F (240°C).

To prepare the peppers, first cut off the stem side of each pepper. Slice open the pepper by making one long cut lengthwise down the side. *Note: Do not cut the pepper in half; make sure the slice only goes through one side.* Use a spoon to scrape out the seeds and veins. Set the peppers aside on a plate or platter.

In a large bowl, add the sausage, salt, black pepper, red pepper flakes, oregano, garlic powder and half of the shredded cheese. Use your hands (I like to use rubber gloves for easy cleanup) to mix the filling until evenly combined. Stuff each pepper with the filling, getting the filling all the way to the tip of the pepper, leaving no empty space.

Add the marinara to the bottom of an 8 x 10–inch (20 x 25–cm) or 9 x 12–inch (23 x 30–cm) baking dish. Nestle the peppers into the marinara, leaving the sliced sides up. Top the peppers with the remaining mozzarella, and cover the dish with aluminum foil, slicing a hole in the center to allow the steam to vent. Place the dish in the oven on the upper rack, and bake for 25 minutes. Remove the aluminum foil and bake for 3 additional minutes, or until the cheese is just melted and bubbly. Serve family-style.

pro tip: Hungarian wax peppers are mild peppers that are perfect for this recipe. But if you can't find them, no problem! You can also use Anaheim, poblano or even regular bell peppers—just cut them in half and stuff them "open faced" to make sure they cook through in time.

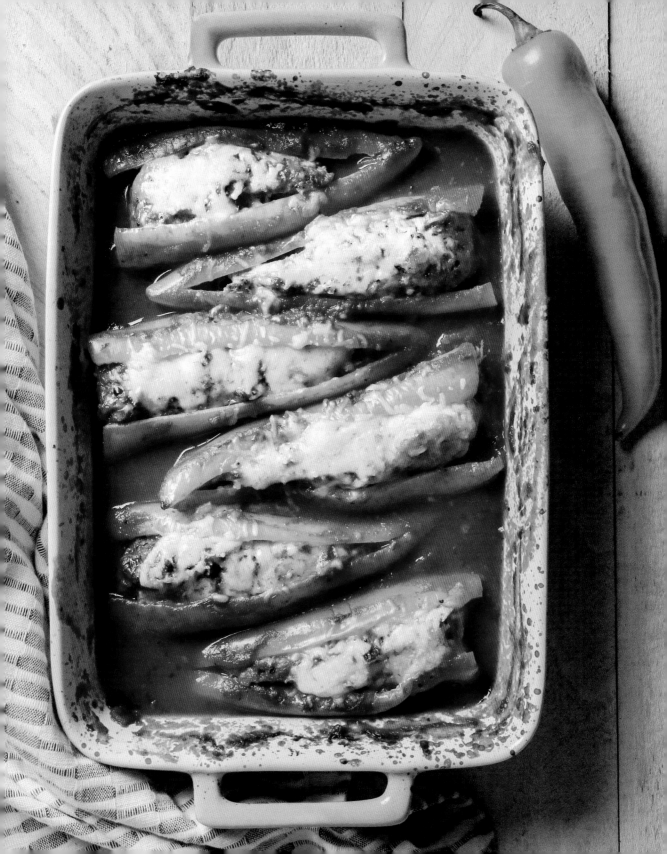

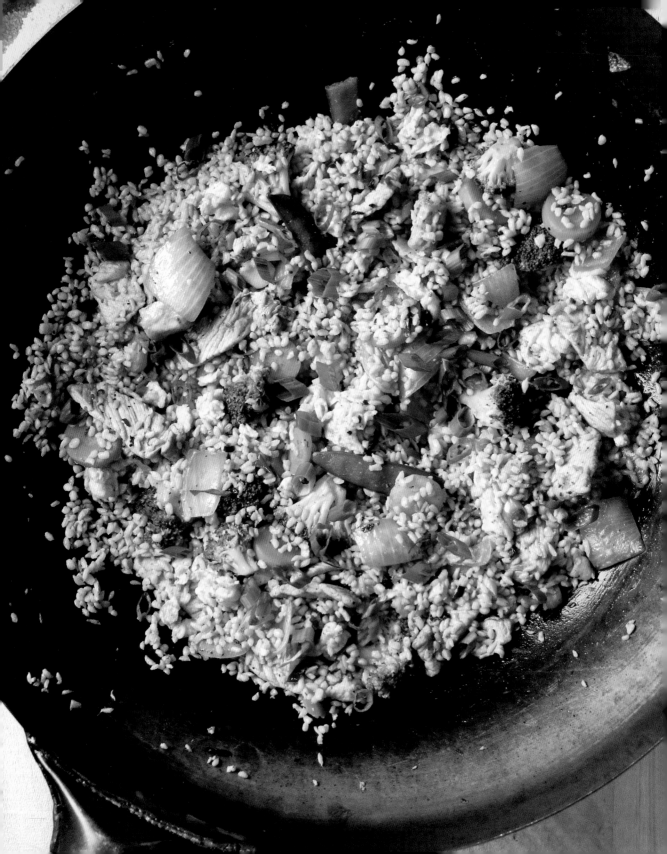

amazing keto pork fried rice

perfect fried rice is hard to come by. But a perfect low-carb fried rice is *really* hard to come by . . . until now! This recipe brings you all of the yummy flavors of your favorite fried ce, but without the carbs. And it's quick and easy to make too. Don't be discouraged by e long list of ingredients. Once you dive in, you'll realize just how fun and simple this ish really is. And I promise you'll be craving it over and over again.

y pairing this with the Blistered Sichuan-Style Green Beans on page 122.

eggs

cup (60 ml) avocado oil, divided

tbsp minced or grated fresh ginger

cloves garlic, minced

yellow onion, chopped

2 oz (340 g) boneless pork chops, sliced thinly

cup (60 ml) low-sodium soy sauce

tsp liquid smoke

½ tsp sea salt

1 tsp freshly cracked black pepper

28 oz (794 g) low-carb rice (I recommend the rice-shaped shirataki by Liviva™ brand; see Pro Tip)

2 cups (182 g) frozen broccoli stir-fry mix, thawed

1 tbsp (15 ml) sesame oil

2 tbsp (30 ml) spicy chili crisp (optional, see Pro Tip)

4 scallions, sliced, plus extra to serve

et all your ingredients prepped and ready to go. Once you begin cooking, it will all come gether very quickly, so having the ingredients prepared is key to this recipe. If you are using a ce alternative, be sure to rinse it extremely well under running water in a strainer, to remove any desirable aromas/textures.

Varm a wok or large (12-inch [30-cm]) nonstick skillet over medium heat. In a small bowl, use a fork beat the eggs. Add 2 tablespoons (30 ml) of the avocado oil to the wok and pour in the eggs. cramble the eggs for 1 minute, or just until they're cooked through. Remove the eggs from the pan nd set them aside on a plate.

ace the same pan over high heat and add the remaining avocado oil. Once the oil is smoking ot, add the ginger, garlic and onion. Stir-fry for 30 seconds, or just until the garlic is golden brown. ir in the sliced pork. Cook for 1 minute, stirring constantly. Add the soy sauce, liquid smoke, salt, ack pepper and rice, and toss. Cook, stirring continuously, for 5 minutes, or until all the liquid s evaporated and the rice turns light brown in color. Stir in the thawed veggies and sauté for minute. Mix in the sesame oil, chili crisp (if using), scallions and the scrambled eggs. Pour the rice to a large bowl, garnish with more scallion, and serve family-style.

pro tip: Spicy chili crisp is an addictingly good, crunchy condiment made of fried chilies, Sichuan pepper and onion. And despite the name, it's not actually spicy; it's just incredibly flavorful. My favorite is the Laoganma brand (look for the glass jar with a red label), which you can find at many supermarkets, Asian groceries or online. It's really worth having this in your pantry, and it gives this dish its special touch. For the rice substitutes, rice-shaped shirataki/konjac rice yields the most rice-like results. Find it online or at your local supermarket. If you can't find it, you can also chop up shirataki noodles into small pieces as a substitute.

serves
4

active cooking time
25 minutes

total time
25 minutes

macros per serving

calories
636

protein
26.4 g

fat
46.7 g

net carbs
6.9 g

active cooking
time
20 minutes

total time
25 minutes

macros per
serving

calories
433

protein
49.2 g

fat
22.2 g

net carbs
4 g

last-minute low-carb "al pastor" bowls

"Al pastor," which roughly translates to "shepherd style," came to fruition when Lebanese immigrants introduced lamb shawarma to Mexico in the 1800s. The lamb was roasted on a vertical, rotating spit. As the Mexican and Lebanese traditions slowly merged the lamb was eventually swapped out for pork and seasoned with the beautifully red colored achiote, a paste made from the achiote plant. Now, tacos al pastor is one of the most iconic street foods in Mexico. Here, this slow-roasted Mexican classic is turned into a quick dinner you can make at home. But the next time you encounter the glowing-red tower of spinning pork, please do yourself a favor and order some authentic al pastor.

Try pairing this with the Fab 5-Minute Spanish Rice on page 125.

quick-pickled red onions (optional)
¼ cup (60 ml) red wine vinegar
¼ cup (60 ml) hot water
½ red onion, sliced very thin

quick "al pastor"
1 lb (454 g) pork tenderloin (see Pro Tip)
½ tsp sea salt
2 tsp (4 g) sweet paprika
1 tsp onion powder

1 tsp garlic powder
1 tsp chili powder
1 tsp dried oregano
2 tbsp (30 ml) avocado oil, divided
1 tsp apple cider vinegar

Cauliflower rice, pico de gallo, cilantro, avocado, cotija cheese, queso fresco, jalapeño slices and/or lime wedges, to serve (optional)

For the quick-pickled onions, add the red wine vinegar, hot water and sliced onion to a small bowl and set aside.

To make the "al pastor," cube the pork into small, ½-inch (1.3-cm)–wide pieces (no need for perfection here). Add the pork to a gallon-sized freezer bag with the salt, paprika, onion powder, garlic powder, chili powder, oregano, 1 tablespoon (15 ml) of the avocado oil and the apple cider vinegar. Seal the bag, removing the air, and use your hands to mix and massage the marinade into the meat. Set the bag in the refrigerator to marinate for a minimum of 5 minutes, or you can let it marinate overnight for even more flavor.

Place a large (12-inch [30-cm]) skillet over high heat. Once the pan is hot, add the remaining avocado oil and the marinated pork mixture, spreading it out in one even layer. Let the pork sear for 2 minutes on one side before stirring—this will help it to form a nice crust. Flip over the pork and let it sear for another 2 minutes. Give it a stir, and then sauté for 1 minute, or until the pork is just cooked through. Set it aside on a plate or bowl to rest. Assemble your bowls with the pork, some pickled onions and any of your favorite add-ins. I like mine with avocado, sliced jalapeño, pico de gallo and cotija cheese or queso fresco.

pro tip: Pork tenderloin is a great cut for a recipe like this where slow-roasting isn't an option. But you can also use the more traditional option, pork shoulder, for this. Just make sure you marinate it overnight. For an authentic Mexican flavor upgrade, add 1 teaspoon of achiote paste or powder to the marinade.

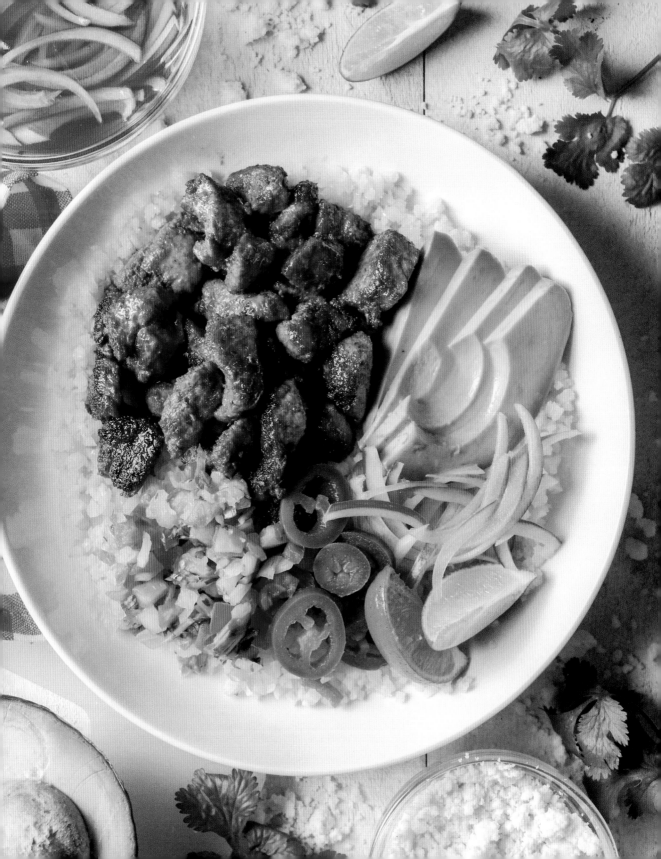

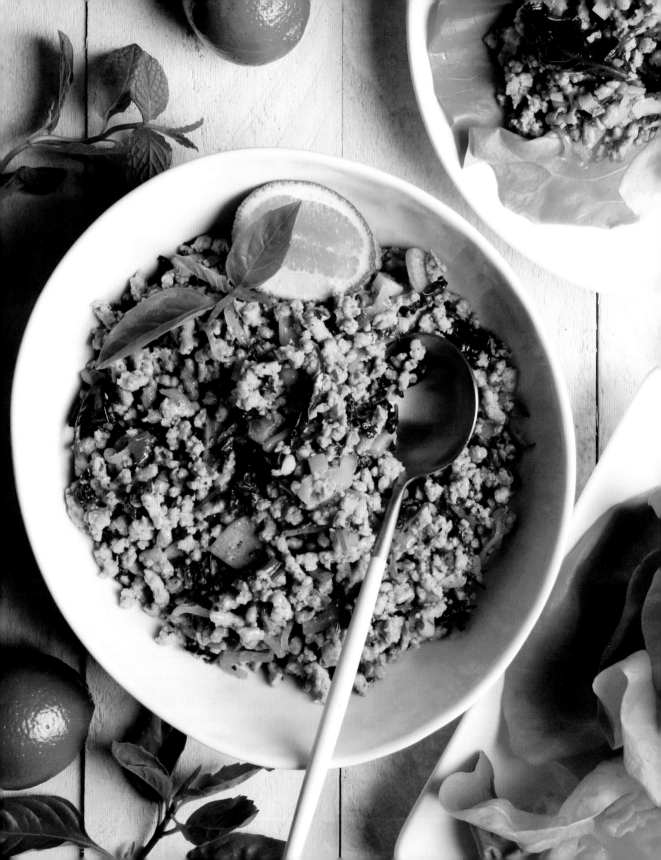

vibrant thai-style pork larb

Larb (pronounced "LAHb") originates from Laos. In fact, it's their national dish. But my mind was blown when I first tried it in northern Thailand. Larb is essentially a meat salad (I mean . . . meat salad? Sign me up!) packed with a bright and tangy sauce and loaded with fresh herbs. As the name suggests, this dish is vibrant and beautiful. And although it normally contains ground rice, I've left that out, along with the sugar, to create a low-carb version that is just as yummy. If you don't eat pork, simply swap out the pork for ground beef or chicken.

Try pairing this with the Thai Green Curry in a Hurry on page 53.

Try pairing this with the Thai Green Curry in a Hurry on page 53.

2 tbsp (30 ml) avocado oil

1 large shallot or ¼ red onion, thinly sliced

2 cloves garlic, thinly sliced

1 lb (454 g) ground pork or chicken

2 tsp freshly cracked black pepper

1–2 tsp (3–5 g) crushed red pepper flakes

2 tbsp (30 ml) fish sauce

¼ cup (60 ml) fresh lime juice (from 3 limes)

1 tbsp (14 g) granulated sweetener (I recommend allulose)

¼ cup (4 g) packed chopped fresh cilantro

3 scallions, sliced

1 tbsp (6 g) packed chopped fresh mint leaves (see Pro Tip)

¼ cup (10 g) packed Thai basil with stems removed (see Pro Tip)

1 head butter lettuce, leaves cleaned and separated

Place a large wok or skillet (12-inch [30-cm]) over medium heat and add the avocado oil. Once the oil is hot, add the shallot and garlic. Stir-fry for 1 minute, or until they are golden brown. Keep an eye out to make sure they don't burn, as this can happen pretty easily. Use a slotted spoon to remove the shallots and garlic from the pan, setting them aside on a plate.

In the same pan, add the ground pork, breaking it up with a spatula. Cook the pork for 4 minutes, or until it's just cooked through, but not yet browned. Stir in the black pepper, red pepper flakes, fish sauce, lime juice, sweetener, cilantro, scallions, mint and Thai basil. Sauté for 30 seconds, stirring constantly. Pull the pan off the heat. Stir back in the fried shallot and garlic, and pour the mixture into a serving bowl. Serve with the butter lettuce on the side for delicious lettuce wraps. This can be served hot or at room temperature.

pro tip: The fresh herbs are key to this recipe. If you can't find Thai basil, Italian basil still works, but don't skip the mint. To me, the mint is what gives this dish its signature aroma.

serves
2

active cooking time
25 minutes

total time
25 minutes

macros per serving

calories
604

protein
32.3 g

fat
48.1 g

net carbs
7.5 g

serves
4

active cooking time
25 minutes

total time
25 minutes

macros per serving

calories
603

protein
56.5 g

fat
65.5 g

net carbs
1.9 g

pork chops in wicked mardi gras sauce

Forget the boring pork chops you've had in the past . . . these chops are here to part
So grab your beads and pour yourself a drink. These pork chops are coated in Caju
seasoning and smothered in a spicy, creamy gravy, loaded with garlic, grain mustar
and a splash of Louisiana hot sauce, of course. And best of all, this yummy dinner com
together in under 30 minutes.

Try pairing this with the Fabulous Bacon-Fried Cabbage Steaks on page 133.

pork chops

2 lb (907 g) thick-cut boneless pork chops

2 tbsp (30 ml) avocado oil

½ tbsp (3 g) Cajun seasoning (I recommend Slap Ya Mama® brand)

½ tsp freshly cracked black pepper

mardi gras sauce

2 tbsp (28 g) unsalted butter

4 cloves garlic, thinly sliced

2 tbsp (32 g) tomato paste

1 cup (240 ml) heavy cream or coconut cream (for dairy-free)

1 tbsp (15 ml) Dijon mustard

3 tbsp (45 ml) whole-grain mustard (I recommen Maille Old Style mustard)

1–2 tsp (5–10 ml) Louisiana-style hot sauce (depending on desired spice level; I recommend Tabasco® or Crystal® brands)

½ tsp sea salt

½ tsp freshly cracked black pepper

Take the pork chops out of the fridge about 15 minutes ahead to temper. To make the pork chop place a large (12-inch [30-cm]) cast-iron skillet over medium heat and add the avocado oil. Seasc both sides of the pork chops with the Cajun seasoning and black pepper. Once the pan is smoking hc sear the meat for 5 minutes on each side, or until the internal temperature of the pork chops reache 140°F (60°C). Pull the pork chops out of the pan and set them aside on a plate to rest. Discard th oil in the pan.

To make the sauce, place the same pan back over medium-low heat. Add the butter and use a whisk scrape the bottom of the pan as the butter melts. As soon as the butter has fully melted, add the garl and tomato paste, and sauté for 1 minute. Stir in the cream, Dijon, whole-grain mustard, hot sauce salt and black pepper. Whisk everything together continuously until the gravy turns red and bubbl Turn off the heat and nestle the pork chops back into the pan. Spoon some of the sauce on top of th pork chops and serve family-style right out of the skillet.

pro tip: If you've ever wondered how some restaurants get their pork chops to be so juicy, the secret is brining the pork. To make a simple pork brine, combine 4 cups (960 ml) of lukewarm water with ¼ cup (72 g) of salt. You can also add flavorings like sweetener, garlic cloves, peppercorns and/or bay leaves. Stir the brine together until the salt has dissolved, then let the pork chops soak in the brine for 1 to 3 hours prior to cooking. This tenderizes the meat and makes it supremely juicy throughout.

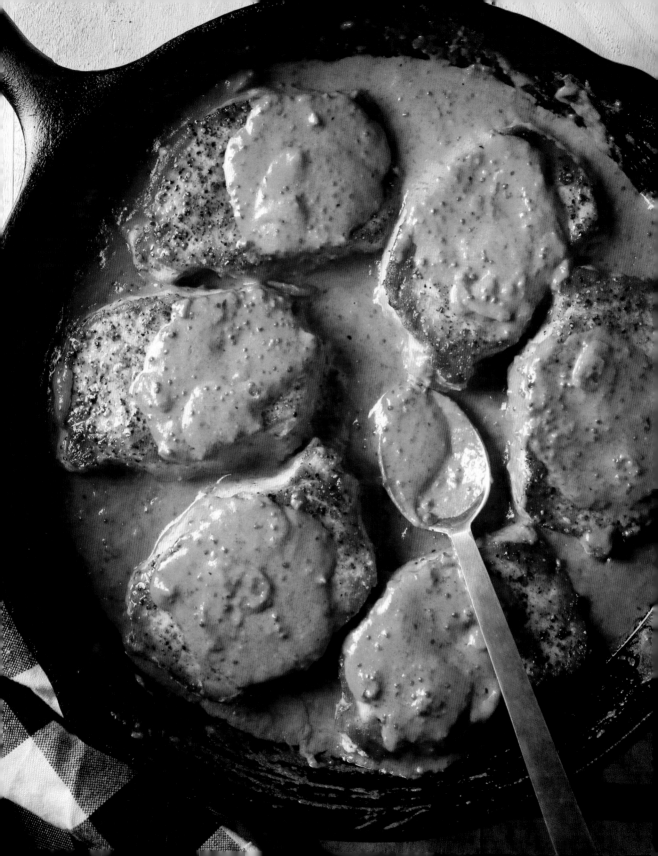

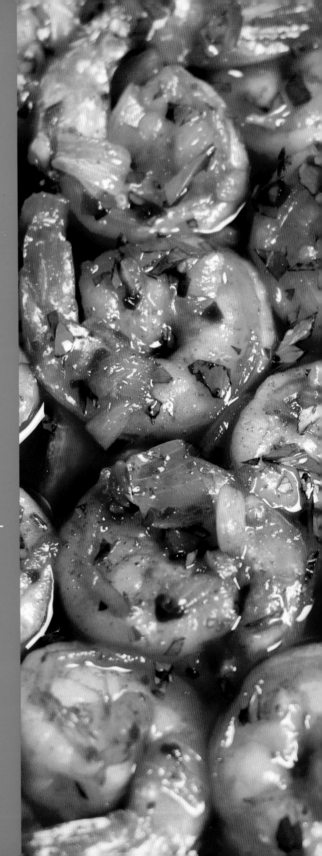

suddenly seafood

You don't need to go to a fancy restaurant to get exquisite seafood. You can make fabulous fish and scrumptious shrimp right at home, and this chapter will show you how. From perfectly crispy salmon to restaurant-worthy grilled swordfish, these are some very special recipes for you to use to impress your friends and family.

Creamy Sun-Dried Tomato Tuscan Shrimp (page 78)

Summery Grilled Swordfish with Avocado Salsa (page 81)

Date Night Spicy Tuna Sushi Boats (page 82)

Kickin' Cajun Shrimp and Sausage Bake (page 85)

Extra-Crispy Salmon and Green Beans with "Horsey" Sauce (page 86)

Luxurious Low-Carb Tuna Pasta with Olive Oil and Lemon (page 89)

Succulent Spanish Garlic Shrimp (Gambas al Ajillo) (page 90)

Lemon Dill Salmon en Papillote (page 93)

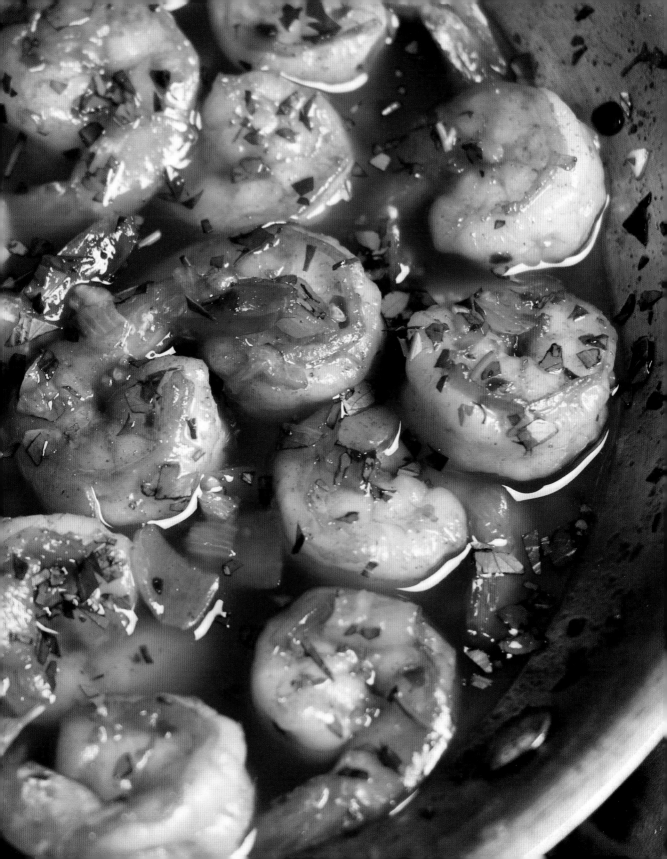

serves
4

active cooking time
20 minutes

total time
20 minutes

macros per serving

calories
508

protein
20.7 g

fat
41.6 g

net carbs
3.1 g

creamy sun-dried tomato tuscan shrimp

Okay, fine. The traditional dish that inspired this recipe is definitely not from Tuscany. But this is one tasty dinner, so I won't overthink it. All I know is, it's good—creamy, rich and comforting. And did I mention that you can make this in 20 minutes, start to finish? If you really want to impress someone on your next date night, make this and spoon it on top of a juicy steak for a mind-blowing surf-n-turf dinner!

Try pairing this with the Simply Delish Sausage and Kale Soup on page 104.

1 lb (454 g) jumbo shrimp, peeled/deveined and thawed (see Pro Tip)

¾ tsp sea salt, divided

½ tsp cracked black pepper, divided

1 tbsp (15 ml) avocado oil

1 tbsp (14 g) unsalted butter

4 cloves garlic, minced

¼ tsp crushed red pepper flakes (optional)

3 tbsp (11 g) drained and chopped sun-dried tomatoes in oil (in the jar)

1½ cups (360 ml) heavy cream or half-and-half

½ cup (57 g) shredded Italian cheese blend or mozzarella

¼ tsp dried basil or oregano

2 cups (60 g) packed fresh baby spinach

¼ cup (25 g) shredded Parmesan

1 tbsp (4 g) packed chopped fresh basil or parsley

Spread the shrimp on a paper towel–lined plate in one even layer, and pat them completely dry. Season with ¼ teaspoon of the salt and ¼ teaspoon of the pepper, and toss until the shrimp is coated with them.

Warm a large (12-inch [30-cm]) skillet over medium-high heat. Once hot, add the oil and swirl to coat the bottom of the pan. Add the shrimp and sear for 2 minutes on each side, or just until the shrimp turn opaque and curl up. Remove the shrimp from the pan and set them aside on the plate.

Using the same pan, lower the heat to medium-low and melt the butter. Stir in the garlic, red pepper flakes (if using) and sun-dried tomatoes. Sauté for 30 seconds, and then pour in the cream and Italian cheese. Stir continuously, scraping the bottom of the pan, for 1 minute, or until the cheese and cream combine into a smooth sauce. Mix in the basil, remaining salt and black pepper, spinach and shrimp. Let everything simmer for 1 minute, or just until the spinach has fully wilted and the sauce thickens. Take the pan off the heat, give everything in the pan one more stir, top with the shredded Parmesan and fresh basil, and serve right out of the pan family-style.

pro tip: To quickly thaw frozen shrimp, place them in a large bowl filled with cool water. Let them soak for 15 minutes. To speed it up even more, change out the water halfway through. And if you peel your own shrimp, don't throw away those shells! Save them in the freezer in a large ziplock bag, and use them to make your own seafood stock for soup. And check out the Secrets of Seafood section on page 156 for more tips on buying and preparing shrimp.

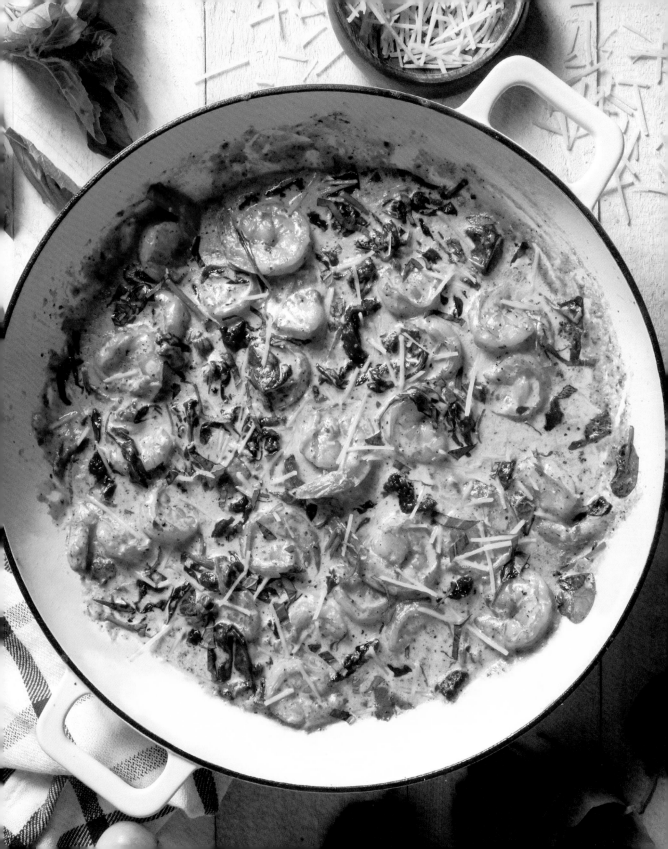

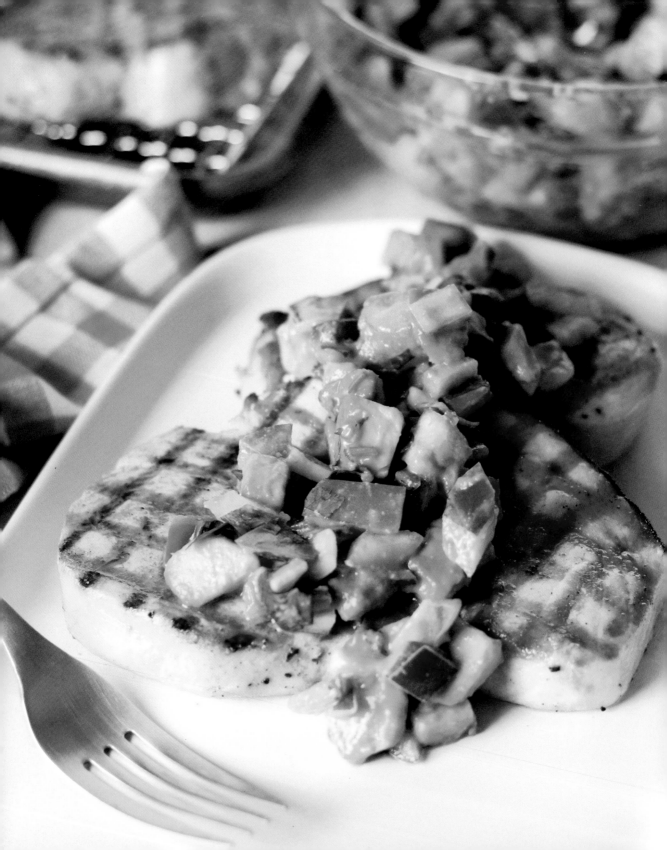

summery grilled swordfish with avocado salsa

Swordfish is such a wonderful fish, but even I sometimes forget to shop for it. It's got an extra-meaty texture that makes it particularly appetizing and really perfect for the grill. It's inexpensive, easy to cook and wonderfully mild in flavor. Once it's covered in this bright and creamy avocado salsa, it just sings! This recipe is ready for summer, and it's packed with protein, healthy fat and beautiful flavor. This works great for any weeknight, but it's also special enough for your next dinner party or cookout. So, fire up the grill, and get ready for these truly delicious swordfish "steaks."

Try pairing this with the Protein-Packed Maryland Shrimp Salad on page 112.

serves
4

active cooking time
25 minutes

total time
25 minutes

macros per serving

calories
439

protein
46.8 g

fat
25.8 g

net carbs
3.6 g

avocado salsa

- 1 Roma tomato, diced
- ¼ cup (60 ml) fresh lime juice (from 3 limes)
- 1–2 jalapeños, seeded and minced
- ½ red onion, diced
- 2 tbsp (2 g) packed chopped cilantro
- ½ tsp sea salt
- 1 large avocado, diced

grilled swordfish

- 2 lb (907 g) swordfish (4 fillets)
- 2 tsp (10 ml) avocado oil
- ½ tsp sea salt
- ¼ tsp freshly cracked black pepper
- ½ tsp cumin
- Nonstick cooking spray

To make the salsa, in a small bowl, add the tomato, lime juice, jalapeños, red onion, cilantro and salt. Stir together until just combined. Very gently fold in the avocado—do not overmix. Cover the bowl with plastic wrap and set it in the fridge to marinate.

To make the swordfish, warm the grill or indoor grill pan over high heat. While the grill warms up, rub the fish with the avocado oil, and then evenly coat it with the salt, pepper and cumin.

When the grill (or grill pan) is smoking hot, generously coat it with nonstick spray, then place the fish fillets onto the grates. Cook for 2 minutes, and then rotate the fillet 45 degrees (for "fancy" grill marks) and cook for 2 minutes. Flip over the fish and repeat on the other side. When the fish is done, set it directly onto serving plates or on a nice platter. Spoon the delicious salsa over the top and enjoy!

pro tip: If you can't find swordfish, I recommend using skin-on red snapper. But halibut, cod, salmon and even shrimp also work great.

serves
2

active cooking time
20 minutes

total time
20 minutes

macros per serving

calories
680

protein
45.5 g

fat
52.3 g

net carbs
7.6 g

date night spicy tuna sushi boats

In my house, date night means sushi, as it is our favorite thing to eat together. But instead of going out, these adorable sushi boats are a fun and interactive way to bring a sushi date night right to your kitchen. And no need to worry about practicing your sushi-rolling skills, as that isn't needed here. Instead, the cucumbers act as the vessel for the spicy tuna filling and give the perfect crunchy bite. So, the next time you want to impress your lover, pour out some sake and make these sushi boats together. Note: You definitely want to look for sushi-grade ahi tuna (or salmon) for this, which you can find in the frozen seafood section at your grocery store.

For dessert, try pairing this with the Seductive Strawberry Mojito Fool on page 139.

2 cucumbers

3½ tbsp (53 ml) sriracha sauce, divided

½ cup (120 ml) mayonnaise

12 oz (340 g) sushi-quality ahi tuna steaks, thawed (see Pro Tips)

1½ tbsp (23 ml) sesame oil

2 scallions, thinly sliced

½ tsp sea salt

½ tsp sesame seeds

Prepare the cucumber "sushi boats" by slicing the cucumbers in half lengthwise. With a spoon, scrape out the seeds in the middle, leaving four canoe-shaped cucumber boats. Set them aside on a plate or platter.

In a medium bowl, combine 1½ tablespoons (23 ml) of the sriracha with the mayonnaise, and stir well to combine. Add the spicy mayo to an empty squeeze bottle (see Pro Tips). Mince the tuna by repeatedly running your knife through the tuna steaks in every direction until the tuna turns into an almost paste-like consistency. You can also dice the tuna instead. Add the tuna to a large bowl with the remaining sriracha, sesame oil, scallions and salt. Stir well to combine. Fill each cucumber "boat" evenly with the tuna filling. Drizzle with the spicy mayo and sprinkle the tops with the sesame seeds. Serve them whole on a nice plate or slice them into bite-sized, sushi-shaped pieces.

pro tips: To thaw sushi-grade fish, place the frozen fish in the fridge 24 hours ahead of time. If the fish is vacuum sealed in plastic, you can thaw it very quickly by placing it in a large bowl with cool water and letting it sit for 15 to 20 minutes.

Don't have a squeeze bottle? Simply use a sandwich-sized ziplock bag. Fill the bag with your spicy mayo, and use a scissors to cut just the tip off the bottom corner of the bag, and you now have a homemade squeeze "bottle" for drizzling the mayo.

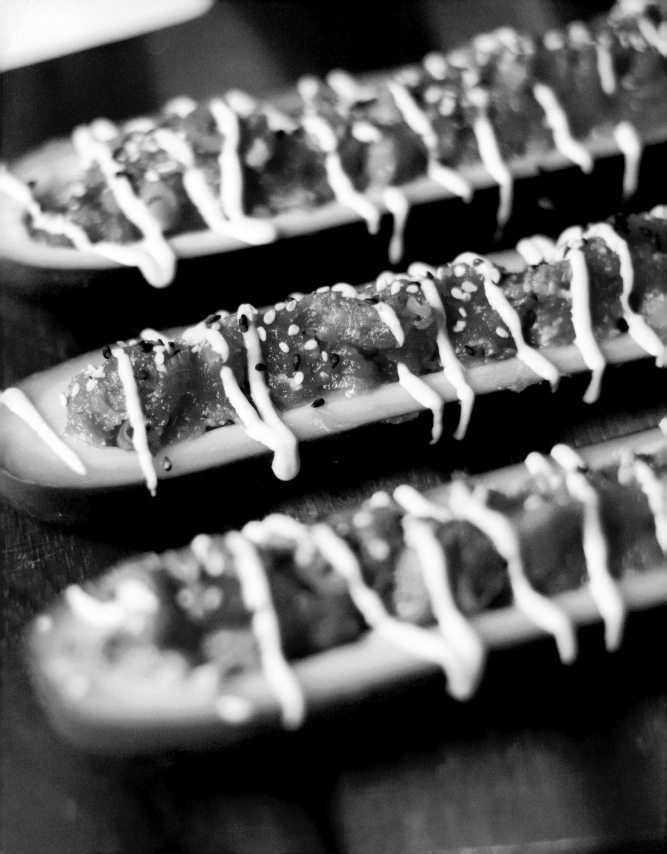

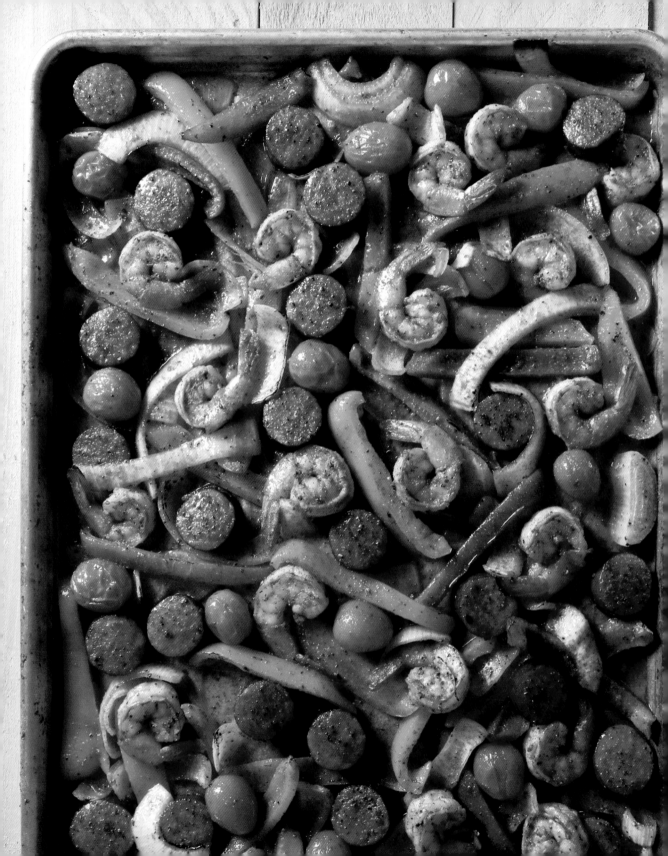

kickin' cajun shrimp and sausage bake

ove a good sheet tray dinner, and this one checks all the boxes. Quick, easy, healthy
nd super tasty, this one-pan meal explodes with flavor. The combination of sweet
hrimp, savory sausage, spicy seasonings and juicy tomatoes is simple perfection.
his recipe has quickly become a regular on the weeknight menu at our house, and for
ood reason.

lb (454 g) jumbo shrimp, thawed and peeled/
veined (see Pro Tips)

2 oz (340 g) andouille sausage (see Pro Tips)

bell pepper (any color), thinly sliced

yellow onion, sliced

cups (298 g) grape tomatoes

cup (60 ml) extra virgin olive oil

¼ cup (60 ml) fresh lemon juice (from 2 lemons)

½ tsp freshly cracked black pepper

½ tbsp (3 g) Cajun seasoning (I recommend
Slap Ya Mama® brand)

1 tbsp (6 g) Old Bay® seasoning

2 tsp (4 g) garlic powder

1 tsp sweet paprika

eheat the oven to 425°F (220°C). Line a baking sheet with parchment paper or aluminum foil and
y the thawed shrimp with paper towels.

ice the sausage into ½-inch (1.3-cm) "coins." In a large bowl, add the shrimp, sausage, bell pepper,
nion, grape tomatoes, olive oil, lemon juice, black pepper, Cajun seasoning, Old Bay seasoning,
arlic powder and sweet paprika. Toss to ensure an even coating of spices. Pour the mixture onto the
aking sheet and spread it in an even layer. Place the baking sheet into the oven on the upper rack
nd bake for 20 minutes, or just until the veggies are tender and the shrimp has curled up and turned
paque. Serve it family-style right off the tray.

pro tips: If your shrimp is frozen, quickly thaw them by placing them in a large bowl
filled with cool water. Let them soak for 15 minutes. To speed it up even more, change out
the water halfway through. And check out the Secrets of Seafood section on page 156
for more tips on buying and preparing shrimp.

Andouille is a delicious sausage native to Louisiana. If you can find it, it goes perfectly
with this recipe. If you can't find it, any precooked smoked sausage will work fine here.

---

serves
4

**active cooking
time**
15 minutes

total time
35 minutes

**macros per
serving**

calories
433

protein
33.1 g

fat
27.2 g

net carbs
6.7 g

serves
2

active cooking time
20 minutes

total time
25 minutes

macros per serving

calories
542

protein
36.2 g

fat
38 g

net carbs
4.4 g

extra-crispy salmon and green beans with "horsey" sauce

I know, I know . . . horseradish and salmon? The audacity! But somehow, this comb just works beautifully. It's bright, fragrant and zesty and will surely make a hors radish lover out of even the loudest naysayer. (Also, did you know that 1 tablespo [15 g] of horseradish contains 44 milligrams of potassium?) The air fryer helps you g chef-quality crispy skin on the salmon in a matter of minutes. If you don't have an a fryer, you can make this in the oven (see Pro Tip), but note that it will take a bit longer. you don't love salmon, this recipe also goes fantastic with steak and chicken.

Try pairing this with the Comforting Keto Cream of Mushroom Soup on page 103.

salmon
2 (7-oz [198-g]) skin-on Atlantic salmon fillets
½ tsp sea salt
¼ tsp freshly cracked black pepper
¼ tsp garlic powder
¼ tsp ground sage
Nonstick cooking spray

herbed green beans
8 oz (226 g) French green beans
1 tbsp (15 ml) avocado oil

¼ tsp sea salt
¼ tsp freshly cracked black pepper
½ tsp garlic powder
½ tsp ground sage
¼ tsp dried dill or basil

"horsey" sauce
¼ cup (60 g) prepared horseradish
2 tbsp (30 ml) Dijon mustard
3 tbsp (45 ml) mayonnaise

To make the salmon, dry off the fillets with paper towels, and then place them on a plate. Season th salmon on all sides with the salt, black pepper, garlic powder and sage. Grease the air fryer tro with the cooking spray, and place the salmon on the tray skin side up. Preheat the air fryer to 400 (200°C). Once hot, place the tray into the air fryer, and cook the salmon for 10 minutes.

While the salmon cooks, prepare the green beans by adding them to a large bowl, along with th avocado oil, salt, black pepper, garlic powder, sage and dill. Toss the beans well until evenly coate with the spices. Once the 10 minutes are up, place the seasoned green beans around the salmon the air fryer tray, and cook the salmon and beans together for 5 minutes. (If you have a smaller c fryer, see Pro Tip.)

To make the "horsey" sauce, in a small bowl, mix together the horseradish, Dijon and mayonnaise When everything is ready, divide the salmon and green beans onto two plates, and serve with th "horsey" sauce on the side.

pro tip: If your air fryer cannot fit all the salmon and the green beans at the same time, cook the salmon first for 15 minutes. Then, remove the salmon and cook the green beans for 5 minutes. Don't have an air fryer? No problem! Simply spread the salmon and green beans onto a parchment-lined baking sheet and roast in the oven at 475°F (240°C) for 20 minutes.

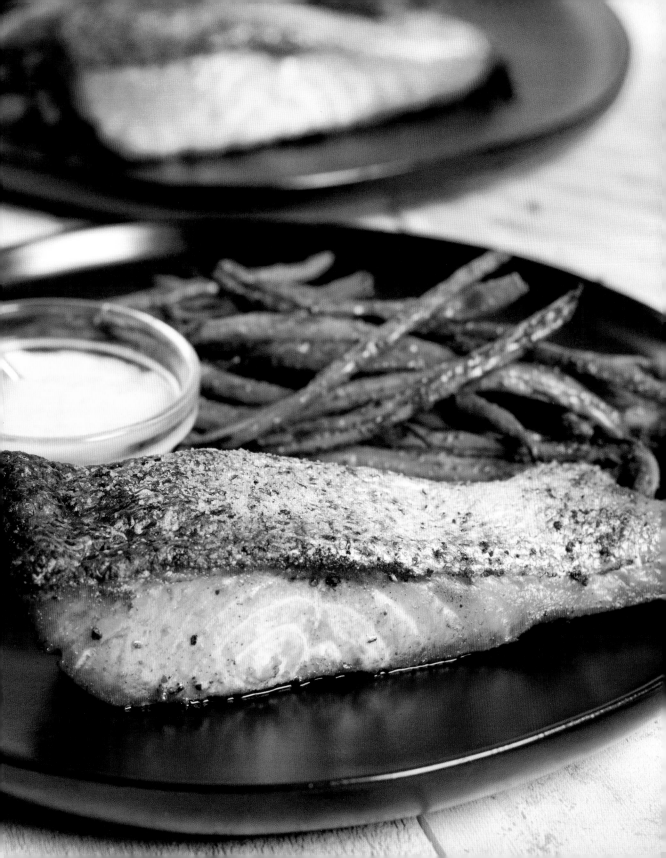

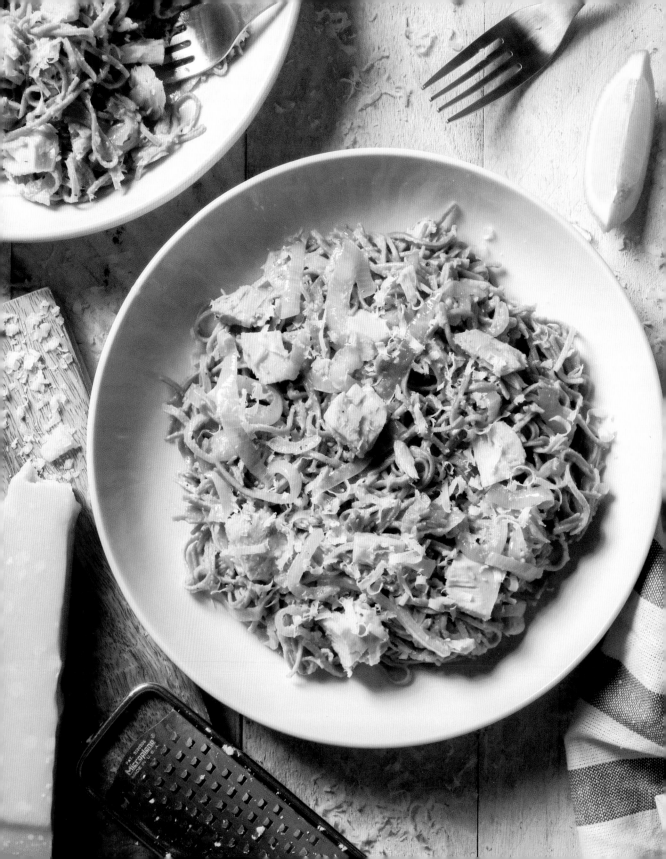

luxurious low-carb tuna pasta with olive oil and lemon

This is the dish my fiancé, Jacob, asks for the most—it's one of his favorite recipes, and for good reason. It's our go-to date night dinner. This warm bowl of pasta is rich yet delicate, comforting yet luxurious, and it uses just a few deluxe ingredients to create something really special. I'm sure that adding canned tuna to pasta sounds a bit bizarre, but this dish uses high-quality imported tuna in olive oil, which is completely different from the canned tuna you may be imagining. Just don't skip out on the aged Parmigiano-Reggiano—it really does make all the difference.

Try pairing this with the Cheesy Baked Asparagus on page 118.

Try pairing this with the Cheesy Baked Asparagus on page 118.

cups (2 L) hot water

¼ cup (57 g) salted Irish-style butter

yellow onion, sliced thin

½ tsp (9 g) sea salt, divided

(7-oz [198-g]) box edamame spaghetti (or your favorite low-carb pasta)

2 tbsp (30 ml) fresh lemon juice (from 1 lemon)

¼ cup (60 ml) extra virgin olive oil

4 oz (113 g) Parmigiano-Reggiano, freshly grated, plus extra for serving

¼ tsp freshly cracked black pepper

3 (5-oz [142-g]) cans Genova® Yellowfin Tuna in Extra Virgin Olive Oil (see Pro Tip)

Fill a large pot with a lid with the hot water. Put the lid on and place the pot on the stove over high heat and bring the water to a boil. Place a large (12-inch [30-cm]) skillet over medium-high heat and add the butter. Swirl the butter around in the pan until it's fully melted, and then add the onion. Sauté for 6 minutes, or until it's translucent and soft, stirring every minute or so. While the onion cooks, make the pasta by adding 1 teaspoon of sea salt along with the pasta to the boiling water. Boil the pasta for 4 minutes. *Note: If you are using another type of pasta, cook according to the al dente directions on the box.*

Once the noodles are al dente, strain the pasta (without rinsing it), and then immediately add the pasta back into its now empty pot. Add the cooked onion, including all the butter from the pan. Add the lemon juice, olive oil, Parmigiano-Reggiano, remaining salt and the black pepper, and mix everything together to combine with the pasta. Finally, add the tuna, including the olive oil in the can, and gently toss the tuna into the pasta until fully coated. Serve immediately in bowls and top each bowl with extra Parmigiano-Reggiano. Buon appetito!

pro tip: Find the imported tuna in olive oil next to the regular canned tuna in your grocery store. If you can't find it, leave it out and make the pasta as written but without the tuna. Instead, top the pasta with seared fillets of tuna or salmon, or even sautéed shrimp.

serves
4

active cooking time
30 minutes

total time
30 minutes

macros per serving

calories
703

protein
54.7 g

fat
45.5 g

net carbs
7.1 g

serves
2

active cooking time
15 minutes

total time
15 minutes

macros per serving

calories
641

protein
31.5 g

fat
54.1 g

net carbs
5.3 g

succulent spanish garlic shrimp (gambas al ajillo)

Perhaps one of my favorite recipes in this entire book, this classic Spanish tapas dish needs little introduction. I could drink up the garlicky sauce with a spoon! This is a true restaurant-quality dish you can make in 15 minutes . . . in fact, I learned it while working at a fantastic tapas restaurant, so this is the real deal. And it's got lots of heart-healthy olive oil, so this recipe is an absolute winner.

Try pairing this with the Blissful Burrata and Pancetta Salad with Summer Citronette on page 115.

---

1 lb (454 g) jumbo shrimp, peeled/deveined and thawed (see Pro Tips)

½ tsp sea salt

½ cup (120 ml) extra virgin olive oil

1 shallot, diced

½ tsp crushed red pepper flakes

6 cloves garlic, minced

½ tsp sweet paprika

2 tbsp (8 g) chopped packed fresh Italian parsley, divided

¼ lemon, for squeezing

Place the prepped shrimp on a paper towel–lined plate, spreading them in one even layer, and pat them completely dry. Evenly season them with the salt, and then set aside. *Note: Get all other ingredients measured and prepped, since once you start cooking, things will move very quickly.*

Warm a large (12-inch [30-cm]) skillet over medium heat. Once the pan is hot, add the olive oil, shallot, and red pepper flakes, and sauté for 1 minute. Mix in the garlic and paprika and sauté for 30 seconds. Immediately stir in the shrimp and cook for 4 minutes, flipping the shrimp halfway through. If you start to see the garlic turning dark brown, turn down your heat (burning the garlic could leave a bitter flavor in the dish). As soon as the shrimp curls up and turns opaque, take the pan off the heat (keep in mind that the oil/sauce is very hot, so the shrimp will continue cooking). Stir in 1 tablespoon (4 g) of the chopped parsley and a squeeze of lemon juice, and serve while it's hot and bubbly. Top each serving with the remaining parsley.

pro tips: If your shrimp is frozen, quickly thaw them by placing them in a large bowl filled with cool water. Let them soak for 15 minutes. To speed it up even more, change out the water halfway through. And check out the Secrets of Seafood section on page 156 for more tips on buying and preparing shrimp.

Upgrade this dish to a veggie-packed, one-pot dinner for two by adding a sliced zucchini or summer squash. Simply add it to the pan and sauté the squash for 3 minutes before adding the shrimp. Then continue with the recipe as written.

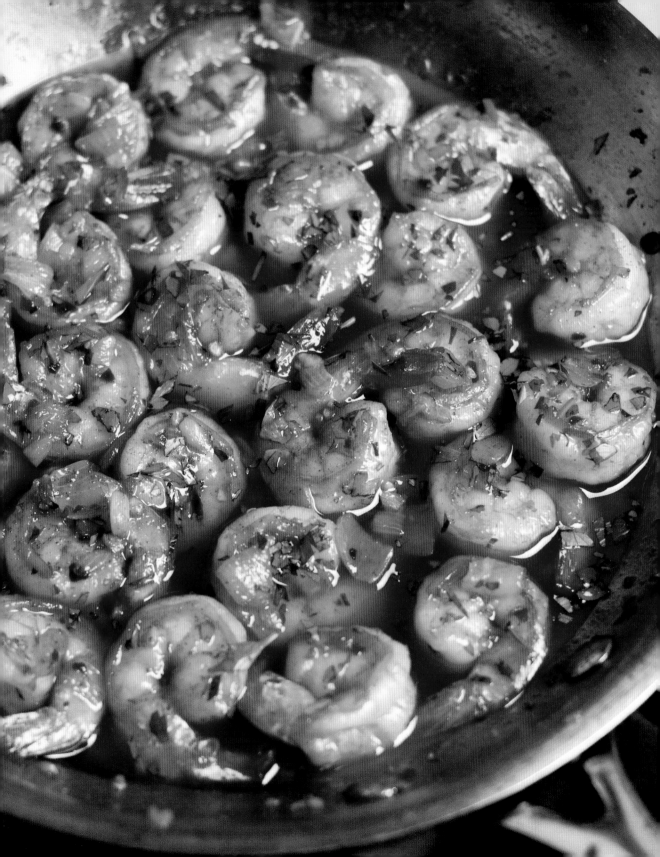

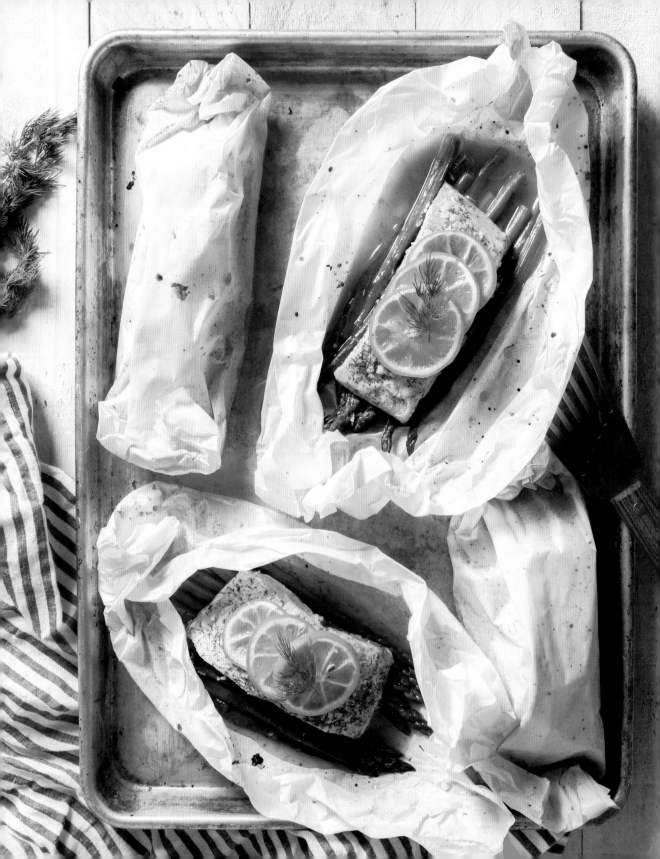

lemon dill salmon en papillote

As a kid, I'd go over to my grandmother's house on the weekends to play Scrabble. She would always make me her lemon fish for dinner—she'd very simply roast fish with sliced lemon on top. So this beautiful dinner, inspired by my grammy, adds a few of my own touches. By wrapping the salmon in parchment, the fish delicately steams with the white wine and lemon. The best part is the "drama" of tearing open those beautiful pouches of deliciousness. I recommend letting your dinner guests rip into the parchment themselves to reveal the gorgeous, fragrant interior. And if you don't like asparagus, try it with any of your favorite green veggies, like broccoli, green beans or spinach. Don't like salmon? Try it with mahi-mahi, cod, tilapia or halibut.

1 lb (454 g) asparagus, trimmed

4 cloves garlic, minced, divided

¼ cup (60 ml) extra virgin olive oil, divided

¼ tsp sea salt, divided

8 tsp + ¼ tsp cracked black pepper, divided

4 (6-oz [170-g]) Atlantic salmon fillets (skin optional)

1 tsp dried dill

2 lemons

¼ cup (60 ml) dry white wine

Preheat the oven to 450°F (230°C).

In a large bowl, add the asparagus, half of the minced garlic, 2 tablespoons (30 ml) of the olive oil, ¼ teaspoon of the salt and ⅛ teaspoon of the pepper. Toss the asparagus until evenly coated. Lay 4 large (12 x 16-inch [30 x 41-cm]) pieces of parchment paper on your countertop. Place the asparagus, divided evenly, into the center of each piece of parchment paper.

Place the salmon fillets on a large plate or cutting board, skin side down, and drizzle the fillets with the remaining olive oil and minced garlic. Rub the oil and garlic all over the top and sides of the salmon. Place the salmon fillets directly on top of each pile of asparagus. Evenly coat the top of the salmon with the remaining salt and black pepper and the dill.

Slice 1 lemon in half. Set one of the halves aside, and then slice the remaining 1½ lemons into very thin rings—you need about 12 rings. Overlap 3 slices of lemon on top of each fillet, almost like roof shingles. Finally, squeeze the juice of the remaining half lemon evenly onto the packets of fish. Carefully pour the white wine around each fillet, so as not to wash off the seasoning. Using the longest sides first, fold the parchment paper up and over the fish, rolling and sealing the edges together. Fold over again on the short sides to completely enclose the packets, pinching the folded edges to ensure a tight seal all around. Carefully place the salmon packets on a baking tray, put the tray in the oven and bake for 12 minutes. Serve the parchment paper packets on plates for each dinner guest.

pro tip: For a fun, spicy twist, brush each fillet with 1 teaspoon of crushed Calabrian chili pepper paste or harissa before placing the lemon slices on top.

---

serves
4

active cooking time
15 minutes

total time
30 minutes

macros per serving

calories
468

protein
32.5 g

fat
33 g

net carbs
3.5 g

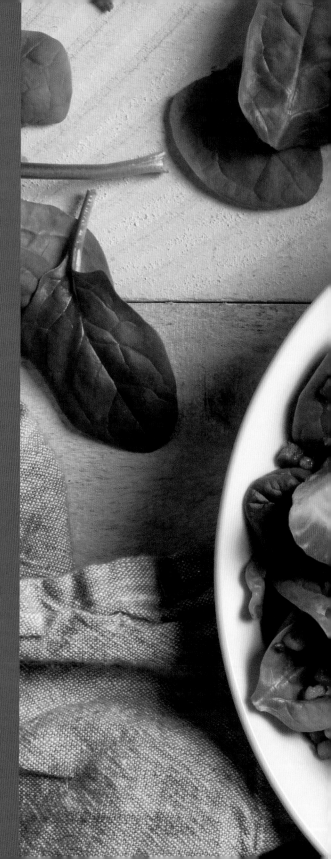

speedy soups & salads

Let me make one thing abundantly clear: These soups and salads are full-blown meals—not dainty side dishes! Could you serve them on the side? Sure. But know that each one of these bowls can stand on their own as a super-charged lunch or dinner. So grab a fork (or a spoon) and get cookin'!

Southwest Roasted Tomato Bisque (page 96)

Easy Egg Drop Soup (page 99)

Hearty Stuffed Pepper Soup (page 100)

Comforting Keto Cream of Mushroom Soup (page 103)

Simply Delish Sausage and Kale Soup (page 104)

The Ultimate Blackened Chicken Caesar Salad (page 107)

Steak and Avocado Salad with Sweet Onion Dressing (page 108)

Loaded Lemon-Pepper Broccoli Salad (page 111)

Protein-Packed Maryland Shrimp Salad (page 112)

Blissful Burrata and Pancetta Salad with Summer Citronette (page 115)

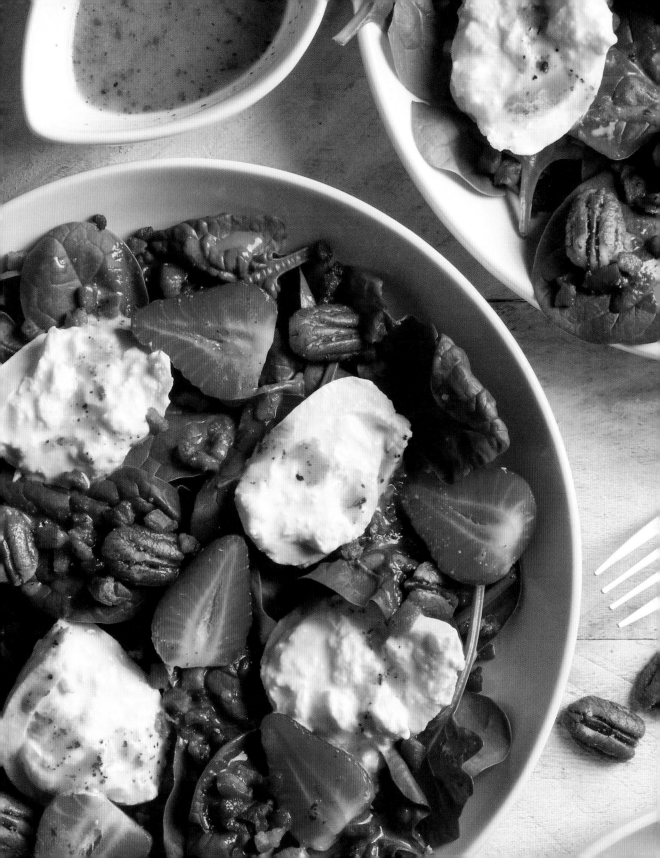

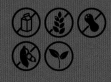

southwest roasted tomato bisque

Tomato soup is a classic comfort food—who doesn't love it with a grilled cheese? Th[
version brings a taste of the Southwest to an age-old classic. Roasting the veggies fir[
gives the soup a subtle, smoky flavor and complexity, while the roasted red peppe[
and spices give it real depth and sweetness. And this healthy recipe is crazy easy t[
make too, with very humble ingredients that yield big results. Note: I love including th[
jalapeño because it gives the soup some fiery heat, but if you don't like it spicy, leav[
it out.

Try pairing this with the Chili-Lime Grilled Chicken with Garlicky Aioli on page 58.

page 58

1–2 jalapeños (optional)

3 lb (1.5 kg) tomatoes on the vine, cut in half with stems removed

1 small yellow onion, peeled and cut in half

¼ cup (60 ml) avocado oil

1 (16-oz [454-g]) jar roasted red peppers, drained

1½ tsp (9 g) sea salt

½ tsp freshly cracked black pepper

1 tsp chili powder

½ tsp cumin

½ tsp smoked paprika

Sour cream or Mexican-style crema, to serve (optional)

Preheat the oven to broil and line a baking sheet with aluminum foil.

Cut the stem ends off the jalapeños (if using), and slice them in half lengthwise. Use a spoo[
to scrape out the seeds from the jalapeño halves. Place the jalapeños, tomatoes and onion cut sid[
down on the baking sheet. Drizzle everything with avocado oil and place the sheet on the middl[
rack of the oven for 15 minutes, or until the skins of the tomatoes are blistered and charred. Take th[
pan out of the oven. Use tongs to move all the veggies from the baking tray into a blender, leavin[
behind any of the juices in the pan.

To the blender, add the drained red peppers, salt, black pepper, chili powder, cumin and paprika, an[
then blend on high speed until the soup is smooth. Leave the blender running for another minute or s[
to ensure an extra-creamy texture. If you have a small blender, make sure to blend it in two batches.

If serving right away, pour the soup directly from the blender into small bowls and drizzle the top wit[
sour cream or crema as garnish, if using. Optionally, you can store the soup in the fridge and serve late[
by reheating it on the stove over medium-high heat until the soup is warm and bubbly.

pro tip: To make this a protein-packed meal, sauté 8 ounces (226 g) of fresh chorizo until it's browned, and top each bowl of soup with a little bit of chorizo.

---

makes
8 cups (2 L) of soup

active cooking time
15 minutes

total time
30 minutes

macros per cup

calories
112

protein
2.2 g

fat
7.4 g

net carbs
6.4 g

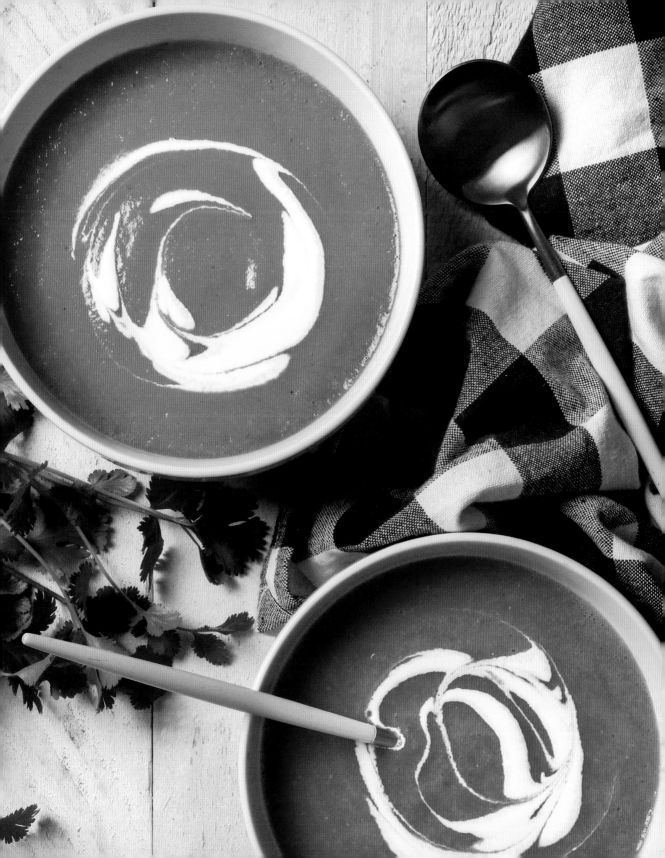

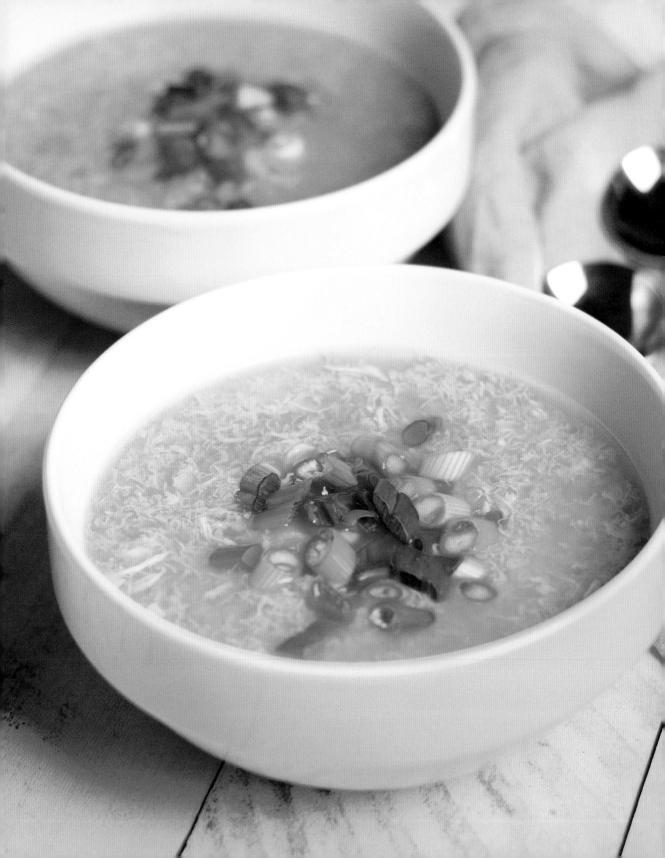

asy egg drop soup

g drop soup is a Chinese restaurant classic, and now you can quickly make it yourself
home! And because the soup is typically thickened with cornstarch, this low-carb
ersion is a bit better for you too. It's also really fun to make and surprisingly easy.
ou'll be wondering why you never made this yourself before.

y pairing this with the Blistered Sichuan-Style Green Beans on page 122.

cups (1.5 L) hot water

eggs

2 tbsp (11 g) chicken bouillon powder
recommend Knorr® brand)

tsp (10 ml) low-sodium soy sauce

¼ tsp turmeric (for color)

¼ tsp xanthan gum (for thickening; optional)

Sliced scallions, to serve (optional)

a soup pot, bring the water to a boil over high heat. In a small bowl, beat the eggs with a fork and
t aside. Once the water boils, add the chicken bouillon, soy sauce and turmeric and stir well. Bring
e mixture to a boil. Hold a colander over the boiling soup with one hand, and with the other, pour
e beaten eggs into the colander. Let the eggs drip from the colander into the boiling broth, while
hisking continuously with the other hand. Hence, "egg drop" soup *wink wink*. Once all the eggs
ave dripped into the soup, let it cook for 1 to 2 minutes, stirring in the xanthan gum, if using. When
e soup comes back to a boil, turn off the heat and stir again. Pour the soup into small individual bowls
nd top with the scallions (if using).

pro tip: Turn this into a protein-packed meal by sautéing 1 pound (454 g) of ground
chicken and adding it to the soup.

makes
6 cups (1.5 L) of
soup

**active cooking
time**
15 minutes

total time
15 minutes

macros per cup

calories
67

protein
3.4 g

fat
2.1 g

net carbs
0.9 g

makes
8 cups (2 L) of
soup

active cooking
time
15 minutes

total time
30 minutes

macros per
cup

calories
302

protein
25 g

fat
17.8 g

net carbs
4.1 g

hearty stuffed pepper soup

This soup is a full meal in a bowl and works great as an entree. In fact, you can mak this a day or two ahead and reheat it for dinner later in the week. It's packed with bee sweet peppers and a hearty broth and really tastes like home. Warm, comforting an delicious, this is a wonderful option for lunch or dinner any day of the week.

Try pairing this with My Big Fat Greek Sheet-Pan Chicken on page 54.

1 tbsp (15 ml) avocado oil
2 lb (907 g) 85-percent lean ground beef
1 tsp sea salt, divided
½ tsp cracked black pepper, divided
1 green bell pepper, chopped
1 red bell pepper, chopped
1 yellow onion, chopped
1 tbsp (16 g) tomato paste

3 cloves garlic, minced
6 cups (1.5 L) beef broth
1 (14.5-oz ([411-g]) can diced fire-roasted tomatoes, drained
2 tsp (4 g) dried oregano
2 tsp (4 g) sweet paprika

Chopped parsley, to serve (optional)

Warm a large soup pot over high heat. Once hot, add the avocado oil. Add the ground bee breaking it up with a spatula. Stir in ½ teaspoon of the salt and ¼ teaspoon of the black pepper. Coo for 5 minutes, or until the beef is just browned through. With a slotted spoon, scoop the cooked be out of the pot and onto a plate. Set the plate aside.

Using the same pot, turn the heat to medium. Add the chopped bell peppers, onion, remaining salt an remaining black pepper into the leftover beef fat. Sauté the veggies for 3 minutes, or until the veggie just start to soften. They don't have to be fully cooked through. Stir in the tomato paste and garlic, ar sauté for 1 minute. Add the beef broth, fire-roasted tomatoes, oregano, paprika and the cooked groun beef. Use a spoon to mix everything together, and scrape the bottom of the pot to release the for (the browned bits stuck to the bottom of the pan). Place the lid on the pot and let the soup simmer f 15 minutes. You can ladle it into individual bowls or serve family-style. Garnish with chopped parsle (if using).

pro tip: For a spicy kick, add 1 teaspoon of Cajun seasoning and 1 to 2 sliced jalapeño peppers! For an extra-decadent creamy version, add ½ cup (120 ml) heavy cream.

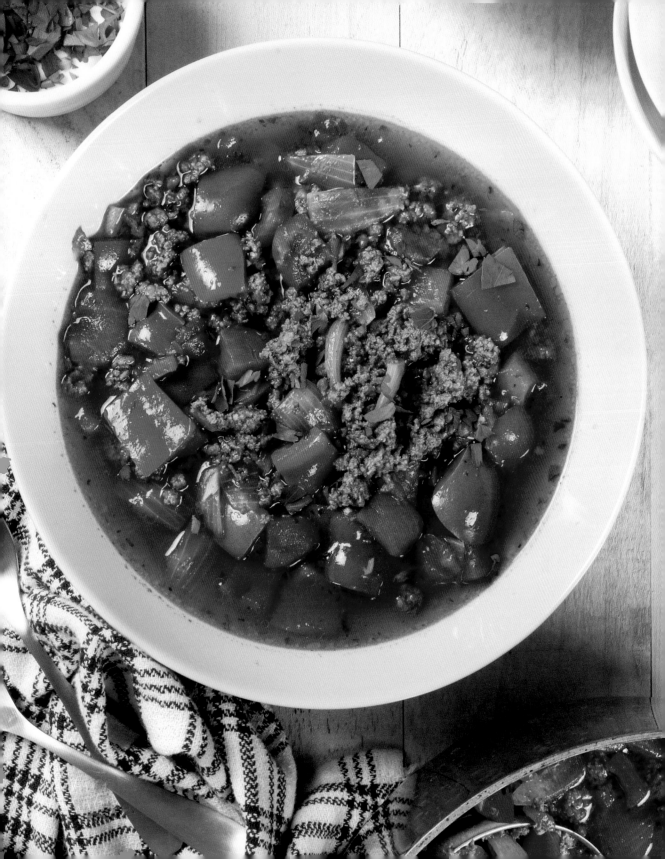

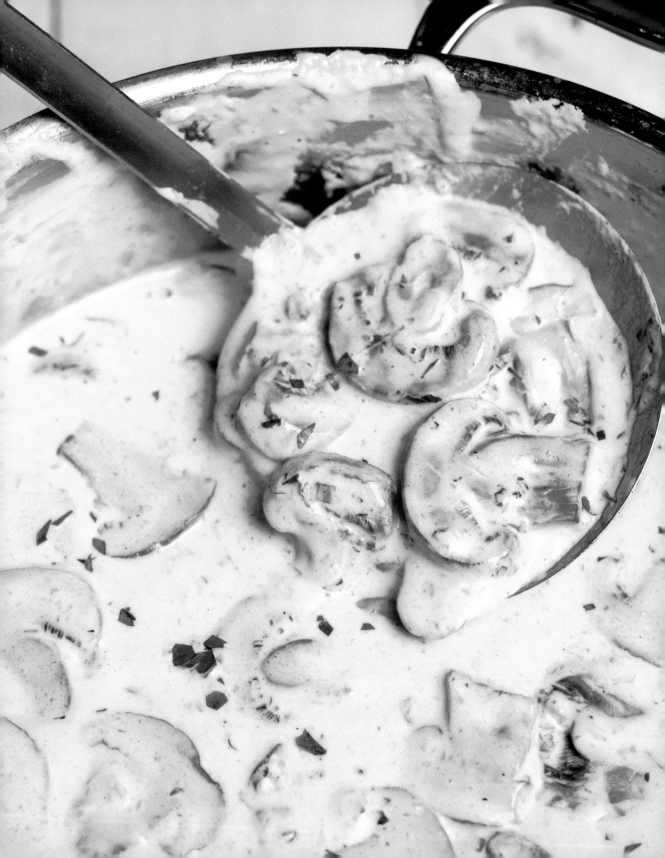

comforting keto cream of mushroom soup

It's finally time we ditch the can of gloppy cream of mushroom soup and make it homemade instead. Not only is it better for you without all the added thickeners, but it also tastes 100 times better too! Rich, creamy and packed with umami mushroom flavor in every bite, this soup is absolutely dreamy. And it works as a starter, side dish or as a vegetarian-friendly entree.

Try pairing this with the 15-Minute Heavenly Steak Bites on page 21.

2 tbsp (28 g) salted butter

1 yellow onion, diced

3 cloves garlic, chopped

1 lb (454 g) pre-sliced baby bella (cremini) mushrooms

1 lb (454 g) pre-sliced white mushrooms (see Pro Tip)

1 tsp dried thyme

1 tsp sea salt

1½ tsp (3 g) freshly cracked black pepper

4 cups (960 ml) beef or vegetable broth

1 cup (240 ml) heavy cream

8 oz (226 g) cream cheese, softened

½ tsp xanthan gum (for thickening; optional)

Chopped parsley, to serve (optional)

Warm a large soup pot over medium heat and add the butter. As soon as the butter is melted, add the onion and garlic, and sauté for 3 minutes, or until they are soft and translucent. Add the mushrooms, thyme, salt and black pepper, and sauté for 3 minutes. Turn the heat up to high, pour in the broth and heavy cream, and stir continuously. As soon as the soup becomes steamy and bubbly around the edges, turn the heat down to medium-low and place the lid on the pot, leaving it slightly open to let the steam escape. Simmer for 10 minutes, stirring every 2 minutes. Add the cream cheese and stir continuously for 5 minutes, or until the cream cheese fully dissolves into the broth. Turn off the heat and whisk in the xanthan gum (if using). The soup will thicken as it cools. To serve, ladle into small soup bowls and garnish with chopped parsley (if using).

pro tip: For an elevated twist, try adding some wild mushrooms to the mix, such as portobello, shiitake or oyster.

makes
8 cups (2 L) of soup

active cooking time
30 minutes

total time
30 minutes

macros per cup

calories
273

protein
9.3 g

fat
23.1 g

net carbs
5.2 g

makes
6 cups (1.5 L) of
soup

**active cooking
time**
20 minutes

total time
25 minutes

**macros per
cup**

calories
259

protein
24.6 g

fat
15.7 g

net carbs
3.2 g

simply delish sausage and kale soup

This is one of those recipes where the soup is greater than the sum of its parts. At its core it's sausage, kale and chicken broth, but it is so, so much more than that. The sausage and veggies add so much depth to the broth, and it really tastes like it's been cooking for hours—yet you can make it in under 30 minutes! This soup feels like something Mom would make when you're not feeling well, and yet also tastes like a restaurant-quality bowl of soup you'd happily pay good money for. You can turn this into your own version of the Olive Garden classic zuppa Toscana by stirring in ½ cup (120 ml) of heavy cream or half-and-half.

1 (19-oz [538-g]) package mild or hot Italian sausage links

2 tbsp (30 ml) avocado oil

1 yellow onion, diced

3 celery ribs, sliced

2 cloves garlic, chopped

½ tsp sea salt

1 tsp freshly cracked black pepper

¼ tsp crushed red pepper flakes

8 oz (226 g) pre-sliced baby bella (cremini) mushrooms

6 cups (1.5 L) hot water

1½ tbsp (11 g) chicken bouillon powder (I recommend Knorr® brand)

2 cups (134 g) packed chopped kale greens (see Pro Tip)

Shaved Parmesan, to serve (optional)

Slice the sausage links lengthwise with the tip of your knife without cutting all the way through. You should just be going through the sausage casing. Peel the entire casing off the links. Cut the links into 1-inch (2.5-cm) pieces, and form the pieces into little meatballs. Set all the balls aside.

Warm a large soup pot over medium-high heat. Once hot, add the avocado oil and the meatballs. Let the sausage cook for 3 minutes, stirring occasionally, until they start to get a little bit of brown coloring. Add the onion, celery, garlic, salt, black pepper and red pepper flakes, and stir everything together. Sauté the mixture for 3 minutes, or until the onion starts to turn translucent. Stir in the mushrooms and sauté for 2 minutes. Bring the heat up to high, and pour in the hot water, chicken bouillon and kale. Stir well. Once boiling, put the lid on the pot, turn the heat down to low and let the soup simmer for 5 minutes. Serve in individual bowls and garnish with shaved Parmesan (if using).

pro tip: If you have a lot of leftover kale, you MUST try my creamed kale recipe. Go to chef-michael.com/recipes/creamed-kale for this recipe and so many more!

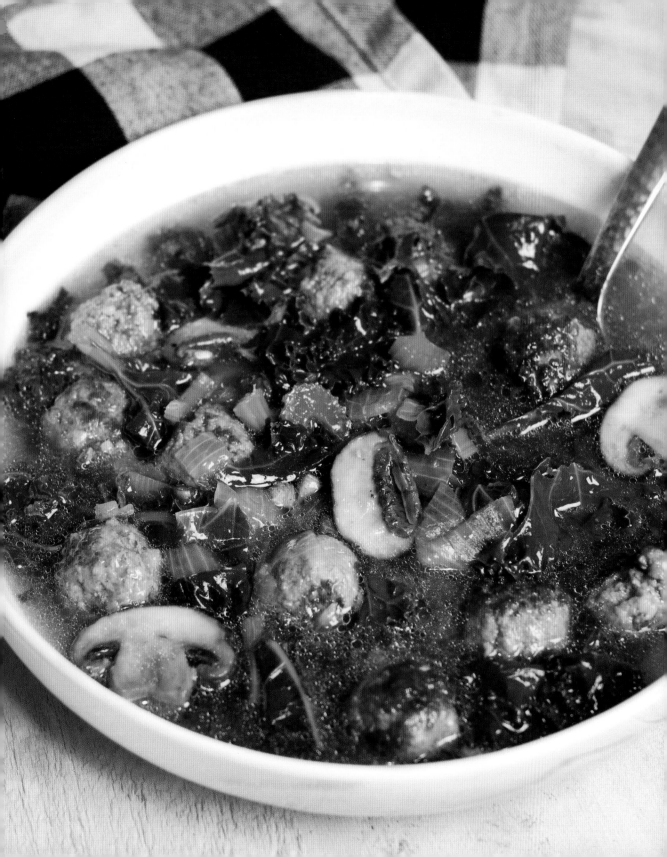

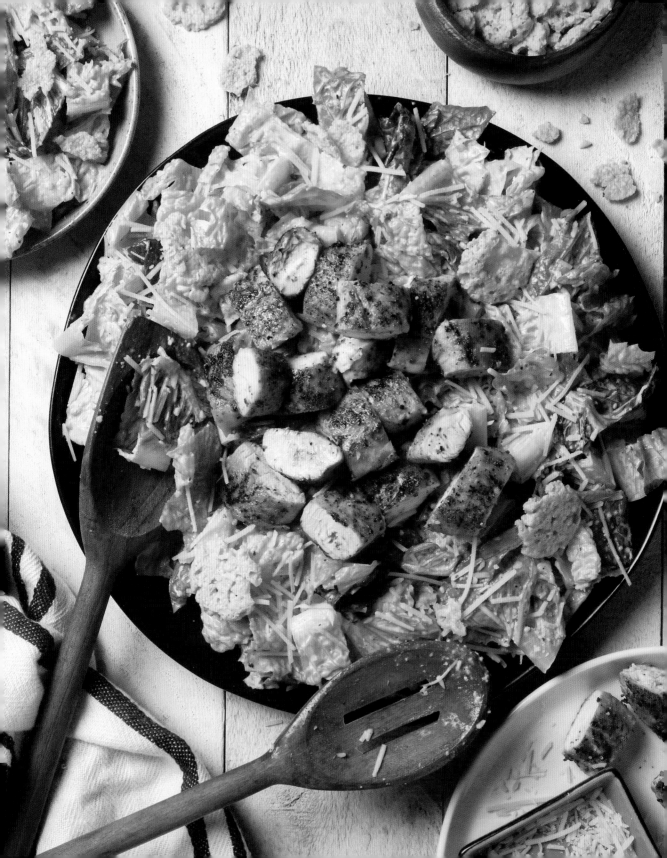

The ultimate blackened chicken caesar salad

This is the restaurant-style Caesar of your dreams! I promise you, this is the best Caesar dressing you'll ever have, so I highly suggest making a double or triple batch. Save any extra dressing in a jar, and it'll last in the fridge for up to 7 days. The blackened chicken in this recipe makes this a protein-packed meal in and of itself, but if you want to use it as a side, try pairing it with the **Quick Chicken Parm on page 50.**

serves
4

active cooking time
20 minutes

total time
20 minutes

macros per serving

calories
333

protein
28.4 g

fat
19.7 g

net carbs
4.1 g

blackened chicken

1 lb (454 g) chicken breast tenders (see Pro Tips)

½ tsp sea salt

2 tsp (8 g) blackening seasoning (see Pro Tips)

2 tbsp (30 ml) avocado oil

salad

2 hearts of romaine, rinsed and chopped

½ cup (50 g) shredded Parmesan, plus extra for topping

Store-bought Parmesan crisps, to serve (optional)

homemade caesar dressing

1 tsp anchovy paste (find it in the canned tuna aisle)

1 tsp Dijon mustard

2 cloves garlic, grated

2 tbsp (30 ml) fresh lemon juice (from 1 lemon)

2 tbsp (30 ml) Worcestershire sauce

2 tbsp (13 g) grated Parmesan cheese

¼ tsp sea salt

1 tsp freshly cracked black pepper

¼ cup (60 ml) mayonnaise

To make the chicken, season the meat on both sides with the salt and blackening seasoning. Place a large (12-inch [30-cm]) skillet over medium heat and add the avocado oil. Once hot, add the chicken and sear for 3 minutes on each side, or just until the chicken is cooked through and the internal temperature reaches 165°F (75°C). Remove the chicken from the pan and set it aside on a plate or cooling rack to rest for 5 minutes, then cut it into ½-inch (1.3-cm) slices.

To make the dressing, in a small bowl, add the anchovy paste, Dijon mustard and garlic. Whisk well until it forms a paste. Add the lemon juice, Worcestershire sauce, grated Parmesan, salt and black pepper, and whisk well. Stir in the mayonnaise and whisk continuously until evenly combined. Place the dressing in the fridge.

Assemble the salad by adding the romaine to a large salad bowl. Pour the Caesar dressing over the lettuce, then sprinkle on the shredded Parmesan. Toss the salad together with two mixing spoons, then place the blackened chicken on top. Serve this up family-style with extra shredded Parmesan and crispy Parmesan crisps on top (if using).

pro tips: For an extra boost of flavor, try grilling your chicken instead. Or, if you're in a hurry, simply use precooked rotisserie chicken cut into cubes.

Make your own homemade blackening seasoning! Simply mix together 1 tablespoon (8 g) of garlic powder, 1 teaspoon of onion powder, 1 tablespoon (18 g) of salt, 2 teaspoons (4 g) of black pepper, 2 tablespoons (14 g) of smoked paprika, 2 teaspoons (4 g) of dried oregano and ½ teaspoon of cayenne.

serves
2

active cooking time
20 minutes

total time
25 minutes

macros per serving

calories
841

protein
50.1 g

fat
64.3 g

net carbs
5.6 g

steak and avocado salad with sweet onion dressing

There's no doubt about it—this is a hearty salad. Juicy steak, creamy avocado and the tangy-yet-sweet onion dressing come together in pure harmony. This recipe is loaded with protein, healthy fat and all the nutritious goodness you'd expect from a beautiful salad. Of course, feel free to double or triple this recipe if you're feeding a family, since this salad is hearty enough to serve for dinner. Note: This also works really well with boneless chicken thighs or salmon as well.

Try pairing this with the Cheesy Baked Asparagus on page 118.

steak
1 lb (454 g) sirloin steak
½ tsp sea salt
½ tsp freshly cracked black pepper
1 tbsp (15 ml) avocado oil

sweet onion dressing
1½ tbsp (23 ml) Dijon mustard
2 tbsp (30 ml) red wine vinegar
½ tsp sea salt
½ tsp freshly cracked black pepper
1 tsp onion powder

1½ tbsp (21 g) granulated sweetener (I recommend allulose)
2 tbsp (30 ml) extra virgin olive oil

salad
4 oz (113 g) baby arugula or spring mix
1 avocado, sliced
1 Roma tomato, sliced
¼ red onion, thinly sliced

Flaky finishing salt, shaved Parmesan, crumbled blue cheese or nuts, to serve (optional)

Prepare the steak by slicing off any excess pieces of fat, and then coat both sides evenly with the salt and black pepper. Warm a large (12-inch [30-cm]) cast-iron skillet over high heat. Once smoking hot, add the avocado oil and steak. Sear for 4 minutes on both sides, or until the steak has a dark crust and has reached your desired doneness (see the Meat Temperature Guide on page 157). Remove the steak and set it aside on a plate or cooling rack to rest while you make the dressing.

To make the dressing, in a large salad bowl, add the mustard, vinegar, salt, black pepper, onion powder and sweetener, and whisk everything together until it's evenly combined. Using one hand to continuously whisk, very slowly drizzle in the olive oil with the other hand, and continue whisking until the salad dressing comes together (see Pro Tip). Set aside 2 tablespoons (30 ml) of the dressing for later, leaving the rest in the bowl.

To make the salad, thinly slice the steak. Add the arugula to the salad bowl with the dressing and toss together until the arugula is fully dressed. Top the salad with the steak, avocado, tomato and red onion. Drizzle the remaining dressing on top of the steak and veggies, and garnish with the flaky salt, nuts or cheese (if using).

pro tip: Instead of whisking a vinaigrette by hand, you can opt to make it in a jar instead! Simply add the dressing ingredients to a clean jar with a lid, seal the lid and shake the dressing aggressively to make the vinaigrette.

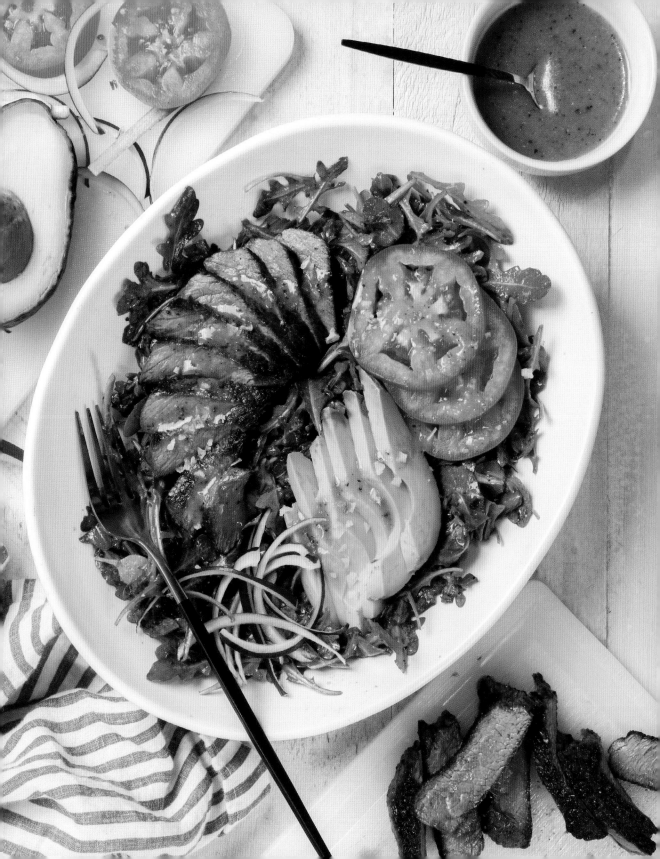

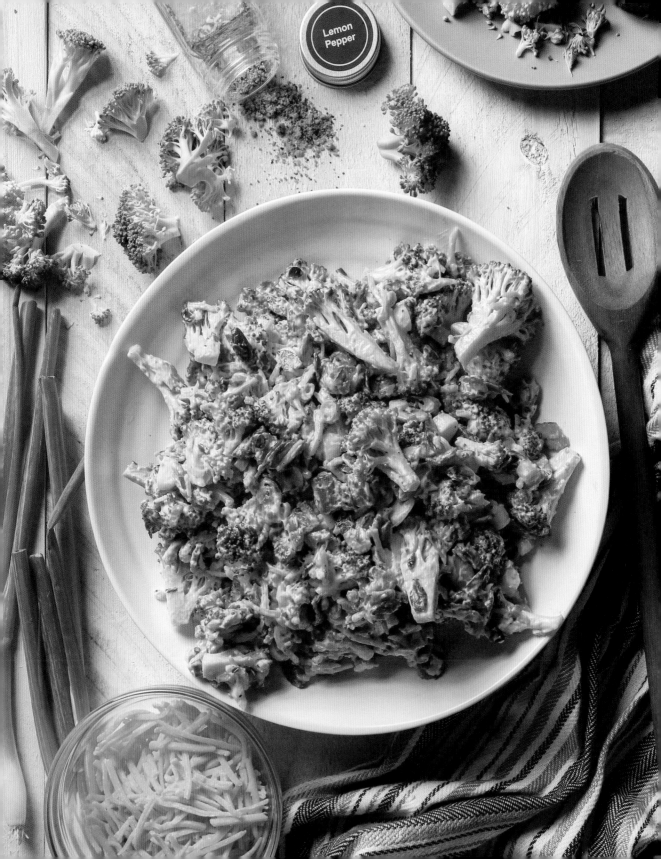

oaded lemon-pepper broccoli salad

ove over, coleslaw and potato salad—broccoli salad has arrived! And this version is aving the rest behind. Fully loaded with bacon, Cheddar, scallions, almonds and the sty lemon-pepper seasoning, this is the only broccoli salad recipe you'll ever need. also happens to be very Keto-friendly and low-carb, packed with healthy fats and otein. You can make this for your next barbecue, or serve it with chicken, steak or fish. nd you can make it a day or two ahead, since it only gets better in the fridge.

y pairing this with The Perfect Garlic Parmesan Wings on page 42.

y pairing this with The Perfect Garlic Parmesan Wings on page 42.

cup (27 g) sliced almonds

2 oz (340 g) bacon, cut into ½" (1.3-cm) eces

(1-lb [454-g]) head broccoli, cut into small rets (see Pro Tip)

1 cup (113 g) shredded Cheddar cheese

4 scallions, sliced

1 cup (240 ml) mayonnaise

1½ tbsp (7 g) lemon-pepper seasoning

½ tsp freshly cracked black pepper

ast the almonds in a dry, large nonstick pan over medium-high heat for 1 minute, or until they turn light olden brown. *Note: Keep your eye on these, as they can burn very easily.* You can also do this in a aster oven. Take the almonds out of the pan and set them aside on a plate to cool. In the same pan, dd the bacon and cook over medium heat for 6 to 8 minutes, or until the bacon is crispy. Remove the acon from the pan and set it aside on a plate. Pour the remaining bacon grease from the pan into a owl to cool. (Do not throw it away!)

a large bowl, add the broccoli, Cheddar, scallions, mayonnaise, lemon-pepper and black pepper. ir the mixture until the broccoli is evenly coated. Add the bacon, almonds and 2 to 4 tablespoons (30 60 ml) of the bacon grease (depending on how "bacon-y" you want it). Stir it together well. I like to t it marinate, covered, in the fridge before serving, but you can absolutely eat it right away. However, gets exponentially more delicious after a day in the fridge.

pro tip: You'll notice that this recipe uses raw broccoli, which gives the salad a lovely, crunchy texture. But, if you like your broccoli tender, blanch the florets in boiling water for 1 minute. Then, dry them off completely before using them in this recipe.

serves
6

active cooking time
20 minutes

total time
25 minutes

macros per serving

calories
459

protein
14.8 g

fat
41.9 g

net carbs
4.1 g

protein-packed maryland shrimp salad

I grew up in Maryland where Old Bay seasoning was born. And we Marylanders swea[r] by it—it's in our blood! We put it on fries, chips, seafood, soup and, most famousl[y] on crabs. (In fact, don't miss the crab cake recipe in my first book, *New Keto Cookin[g]*[.] **Gordon Ramsay called them "Top 10 in the world.") This shrimp salad is a perfect wa[y] to bring seafood to your menu. And to make it even easier, you can make it a day o[r] two ahead—it only gets better marinating in the fridge. It works great as a side dish o[r] as the main entree, so pack it for lunch, use it for meal prepping or serve it for dinner.**

serves
4

active cooking time
25 minutes

total time
25 minutes

macros per serving

calories
349

protein
31.4 g

fat
20.8 g

net carbs
0.7 g

8 cups (2 L) hot water

¼ cup (13 g) minced packed fresh dill, plus extra for garnish

½ cup (120 ml) mayonnaise

2 tbsp (30 ml) whole-grain mustard (I recommend Maille Old Style)

1 tbsp (6 g) Old Bay seasoning

⅛ tsp freshly cracked black pepper

2 lb (907 g) large shrimp, peeled/deveined an[d] thawed (see Pro Tip)

In a large, lidded pot, bring the water to a boil over high heat. While the water heats up, to a larg[e] bowl, add the dill, mayonnaise, mustard, Old Bay and black pepper. Mix everything together wel[l.] Once the water is at a rolling boil, drop in the shrimp and put the lid on the pot. Cook the shrimp fo[r] 3 minutes, or until the shrimp are curled up and opaque. Strain the shrimp in a colander, and the[n] immediately run cold water over the shrimp to stop the cooking. Let the cold water run for at lea[st] 2 minutes, tossing the shrimp every few seconds, to completely cool the shrimp. (This is also a goo[d] time to check for any shells that accidentally made it into the batch.) *Note: You do not want the shrim[p] hot when you mix the salad together.*

Line a large plate with a double layer of paper towels. Pour the cooled shrimp onto the paper towel[s] and pat them completely dry. Add the shrimp to the bowl with the mayonnaise mixture. Using a spatul[a] or spoon, mix everything together until well combined and evenly coated. You can serve the sala[d] right away by plating it in a nice serving bowl and garnishing with the fresh dill. Or store it in a seale[d] container for up to 3 days in the fridge.

pro tip: If you're in a hurry, you can absolutely make this dish using precooked shrimp instead of raw. Just make sure they are thawed and dried off before stirring them into the mayo and spice mixture. To quickly thaw frozen shrimp, place them in a large bowl filled with cool water. Let them soak for 15 minutes. To speed it up even more, change out the water halfway through. And if you peel your own shrimp, don't throw away those shells! Save them in the freezer in a large ziplock bag, and use them to make your own seafood stock for soup. And check out the Secrets of Seafood section on page 156 for more tips on buying and preparing shrimp.

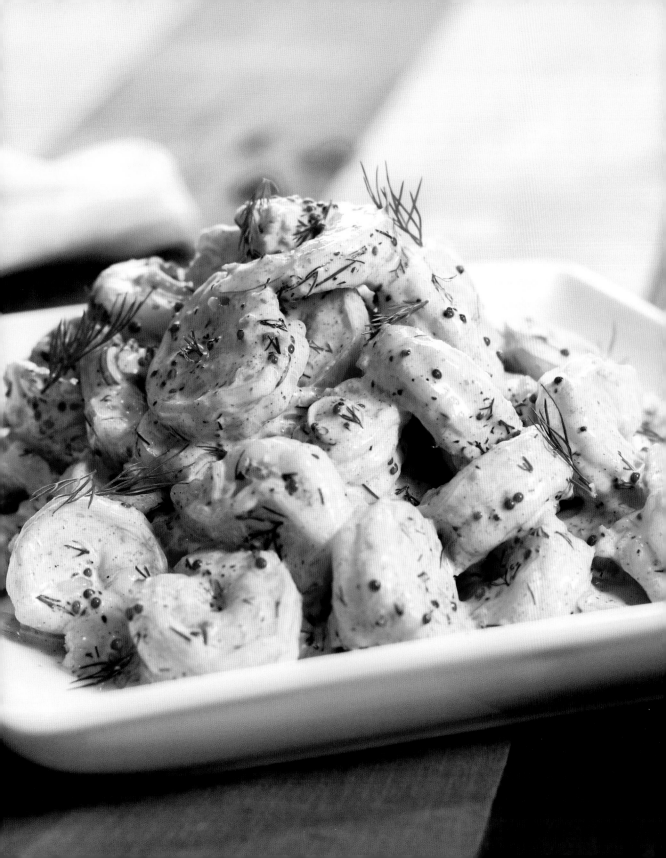

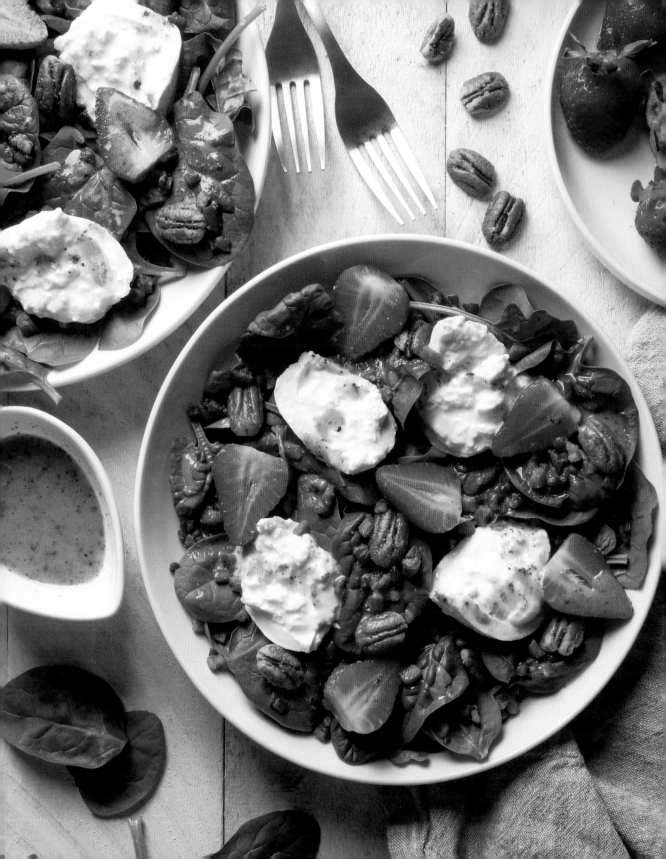

blissful burrata and pancetta salad with summer citronette

Creamy burrata, crispy pancetta, sweet strawberries and a refreshing citrus dressing? This is definitely a salad to impress. It's a restaurant-quality salad you can easily serve for a date night or dinner party, yet easy enough to make for just yourself for a delicious lunch (#treatyourself, amirite?). And the homemade citrus dressing is simply delightful as it bursts with fresh orange and lemon. Fun fact: This dressing is called a citronette, not a vinaigrette, as it uses citrus instead of vinegar as the acid in the dressing.

Try pairing this with the Zesty "Honey Mustard" Chicken on page 46.

Try pairing this with the Zesty "Honey Mustard" Chicken on page 46.

serves
2

active cooking time
15 minutes

total time
20 minutes

macros per serving

calories
569

protein
27 g

fat
42.9 g

net carbs
7.8 g

summer citronette (see pro tips)

Juice from ½ navel orange

Zest from ½ navel orange

2 tbsp (30 ml) fresh lemon juice (from 1 lemon)

1½ tbsp (23 ml) Dijon mustard

¼ tsp sea salt

½ tsp freshly cracked black pepper

1 tsp dried basil or 1 tbsp (2 g) chopped fresh basil

1 tsp granulated sweetener (I recommend allulose)

1 tbsp (15 ml) extra virgin olive oil

burrata and pancetta salad

2 oz (57 g) chopped pancetta or bacon

4 oz (113 g) baby spinach or spring mix

2 fresh strawberries, sliced

¼ cup (29 g) salted pecan halves (optional)

8 oz (226 g) burrata cheese or fresh mozzarella

To make the citronette, in a small jar with a lid, add the orange juice, zest, lemon juice, mustard, salt, black pepper, basil, sweetener and olive oil. Close the lid, and aggressively shake the jar for 30 seconds, or until the dressing is fully combined and creamy. Set the dressing aside in the fridge.

To make the salad, in a small frying pan over medium heat, add the pancetta and sauté it for 5 minutes, or until it gets crispy. Make sure to stir every minute or so. Scoop it out of the pan and place it onto a paper towel–lined plate to drain. Assemble the salad by dividing the spinach evenly into two large salad bowls. Place the strawberries, pecans (if using) and burrata on top. (I suggest slicing the burrata in half once it's on the salad to reveal its creamy interior.) Sprinkle the tops of the salads with the crispy pancetta and drizzle on the citronette.

pro tips: You can also make this citronette with grapefruit or Meyer lemon instead of orange, for a more floral flavor.

Add any of your favorite summery toppings to this! Try it with tomatoes, peppers, blueberries or blackberries, or swap the pecans for cashews or shelled pistachios.

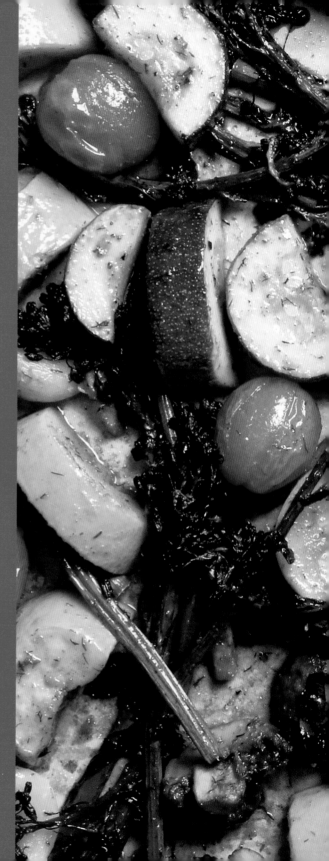

standout sides

Even in a hurry, you can make a full spread for dinner—sides and all. But be careful, because these sides are so good, they'll steal the show! These quick veggies are easy to make and are unapologetically packed with fabulous flavors.

Cheesy Baked Asparagus (page 118)

Sweet Balsamic-Glazed Brussels (page 121)

Blistered Sichuan-Style Green Beans (page 122)

Fab 5-Minute Spanish Rice (page 125)

Herby Pan-Roasted Mushrooms (page 126)

Beautifully Layered Eggplant Caprese (page 129)

Lemony Spice-Roasted Mixed Veggies (page 130)

Fabulous Bacon-Fried Cabbage Steaks (page 133)

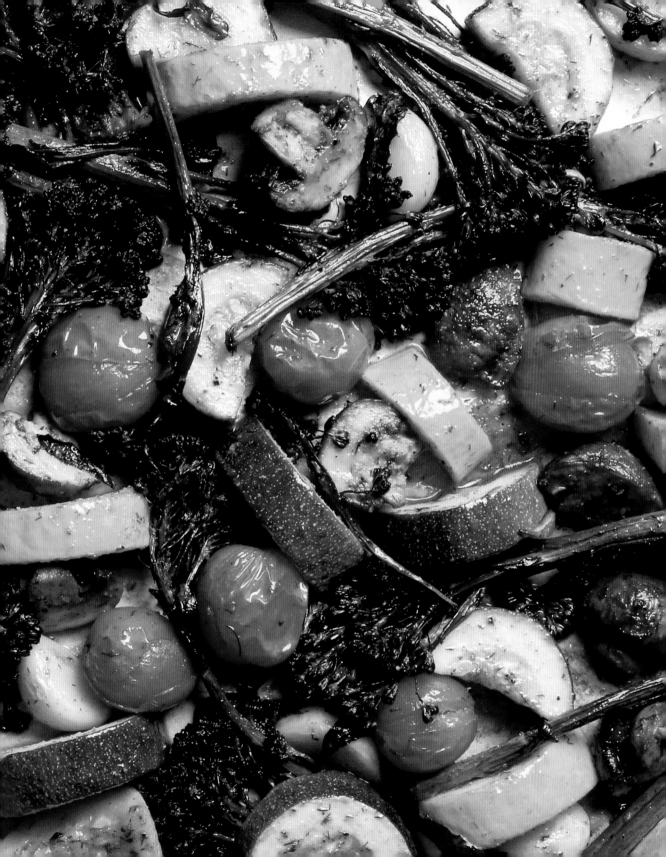

cheesy baked asparagus

Look, I'm warning you now: Make a double batch of this recipe. Your dish will be empty before the rest of dinner is even served. For a big family? Triple it! This recipe is so easy it's perfect for any weeknight, but fancy (and tasty) enough even for the holidays. Who knew asparagus could be so divine?

Try pairing this with the Zesty "Honey Mustard" Chicken on page 46.

Try pairing this with the Zesty "Honey Mustard" Chicken on page 46.

1 lb (454 g) asparagus, stems trimmed (see Pro Tip)

¼ cup (60 ml) heavy cream or half-and-half

1 clove garlic, minced

¼ tsp sea salt

¼ tsp freshly cracked black pepper

¼ tsp Italian herb blend

2 tbsp (13 g) grated Parmesan, divided

½ cup (56 g) shredded Italian cheese blend or mozzarella

Preheat the oven to 450°F (230°C).

In a baking dish, add the asparagus, heavy cream, garlic, salt, black pepper, Italian herb blend and 1 tablespoon (7 g) of the Parmesan. Use your hands or tongs to gently toss the asparagus in the cream and herbs until evenly coated. Arrange the asparagus in one, flat layer, and top just across the center of the asparagus with the shredded cheese. Bake for 20 minutes. Sprinkle the remaining Parmesan over the top and serve family-style.

pro tip: Don't like asparagus? This also works great with broccoli, cauliflower, Brussels sprouts or green beans.

---

macros per serving

calories
131

protein
8.1 g

fat
10.3 g

net carbs
4 g

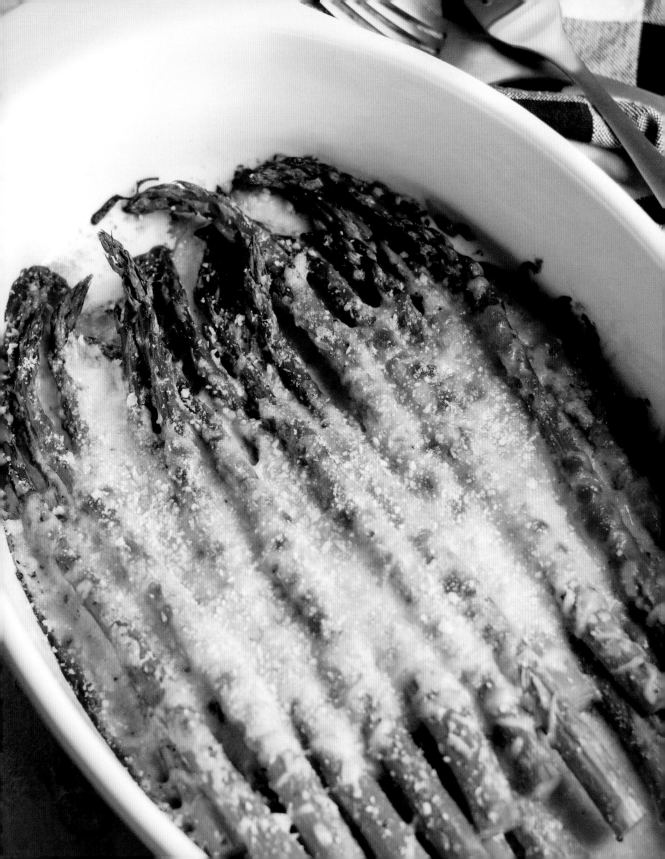

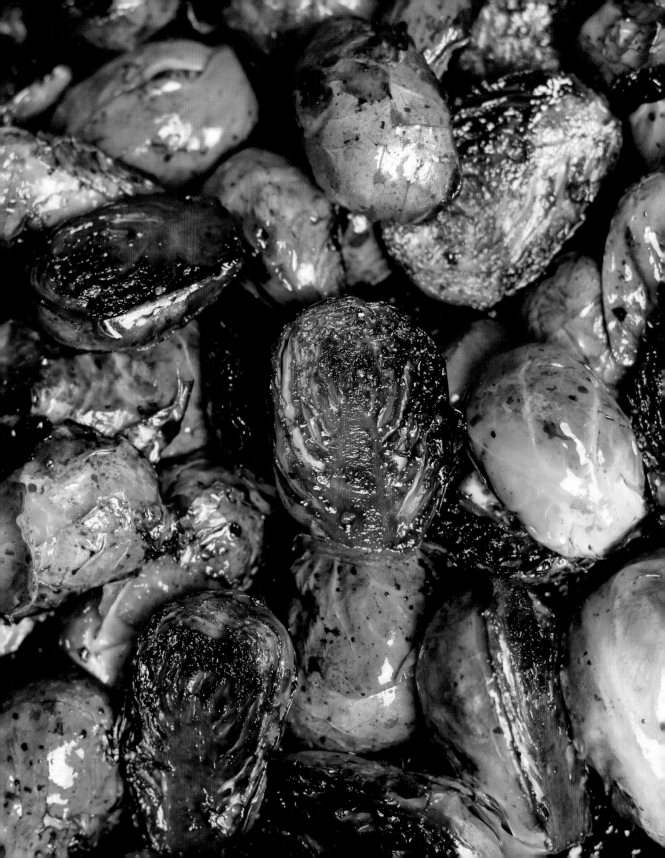

sweet balsamic-glazed brussels

Sweet, salty and tangy, these sprouts are ready to shine! And they get really nicely caramelized and crispy in the balsamic as it reduces and gets almost sticky. Heck, you might even be able to get your kids to eat these green bites of goodness.

Try pairing this with the 15-Minute Heavenly Steak Bites on page 21.

2 tbsp (30 ml) avocado oil

½ tsp sea salt

¼ tsp freshly cracked black pepper

½ tsp garlic powder

1 tbsp (14 g) granulated sweetener (I recommend allulose)

½ cup (120 ml) balsamic vinegar

1 lb (454 g) Brussels sprouts, cut in half

Place a large (12-inch [30-cm]) cast-iron skillet over medium heat and add the avocado oil. Swirl the oil around to coat the bottom of the pan. In a small bowl, mix together the salt, black pepper, garlic powder, sweetener and balsamic vinegar until evenly combined. Set the bowl aside.

Once the pan is hot, pour the Brussels into the pan, and with tongs, carefully turn every Brussels sprout cut side down in the pan. Once they are all facedown, don't touch them, and let them sear for 3 minutes. Check to make sure the Brussels aren't burning—you want a slight golden brown color. If they're starting to turn really dark brown, turn down the heat. Slowly drizzle the balsamic sauce all over the Brussels sprouts in the pan—don't flip/stir the Brussels yet—and turn the heat up to high. Let the sauce simmer for 4 minutes, or until the sauce becomes thick and syrupy. Then immediately remove the pan from the heat, toss the Brussels to evenly coat them in the thickened sauce and pour them into a serving bowl.

pro tip: Take this dish to the next level by garnishing with chopped bacon, shaves of Parmesan cheese, sliced jalapeños or even fresh basil.

---

serves
4

active cooking time
15 minutes

total time
15 minutes

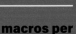

macros per serving

calories
122

protein
3.9 g

fat
7.4 g

net carbs
9.8 g

serves
4

active cooking time
20 minutes

total time
20 minutes

macros per serving

calories
254

protein
3.6 g

fat
22.4 g

net carbs
2.8 g

blistered sichuan-style green beans

I know this is supposed to be a side dish, but honestly, I could eat this whole thing as my meal. It is that good. In fact, I'd call these green beans nothing short of addicting (I suggest making a double batch because you WILL NOT be able to stop eating these!). They are salty, sweet and slightly smoky, with just enough spice and crunch to keep you going back for more.

Try pairing this with Mike's Famous Bourbon Chicken on page 38.

1 lb (454 g) green beans, ends trimmed (see Pro Tips)

¼ cup (60 ml) low-sodium soy sauce

1 tbsp (14 g) granulated sweetener (I recommend allulose)

4 cloves garlic, minced

1 tsp minced or grated fresh ginger

2 tbsp (30 ml) spicy chili crisp (see Pro Tips)

2 tbsp (30 ml) avocado oil

Dry off the green beans with paper towels, then set them aside on a plate. *Note: drying the green beans helps prevent the oil in the pan from splattering.* In a small bowl, add the soy sauce, sweetener, garlic, ginger and chili crisp, and mix together well to combine. Set the sauce aside.

Warm a large (12-inch [30-cm]) wok or skillet over high heat. Once smoking hot, add the oil and green beans, and toss with tongs until the green beans are fully coated. Spread the beans out in an even layer in the pan, and without moving them, let them char or blister for 2 minutes. Toss them again and repeat the char three more times, for a total cook time of 8 minutes. The green beans should be wrinkly with dark blister marks. Take the beans out of the pan and set them aside on a platter.

Place the same skillet back over high heat and pour in the sauce. Once the sauce is boiling, lower the heat and let it simmer, stirring occasionally, for 5 minutes, or until the liquid reduces to a thick sauce. Toss the green beans back in and coat them completely in that amazing sauce. Continue stir-frying the beans for 1 minute, or just until the majority of the liquid has evaporated from the bottom of the pan. Pour the green beans onto a large plate or bowl and serve family-style (silverware optional!).

pro tips: To save time, I buy my green beans prewashed and trimmed in the bag from the produce department. You can also turn this into a protein-packed entree by sautéing 1 pound (454 g) of ground pork before adding the sauce to the pan.

Spicy chili crisp is an addictingly good, crunchy condiment made of fried chilies, Sichuan pepper and onion. It adds flavor and texture to just about any dish. And despite the name, it's not actually spicy; it's just incredibly flavorful. My favorite is the Laoganma brand (look for the glass jar with a red label), which you can find at many supermarkets, Asian groceries or online. It's really worth having this in your pantry, and it gives this dish its special touch.

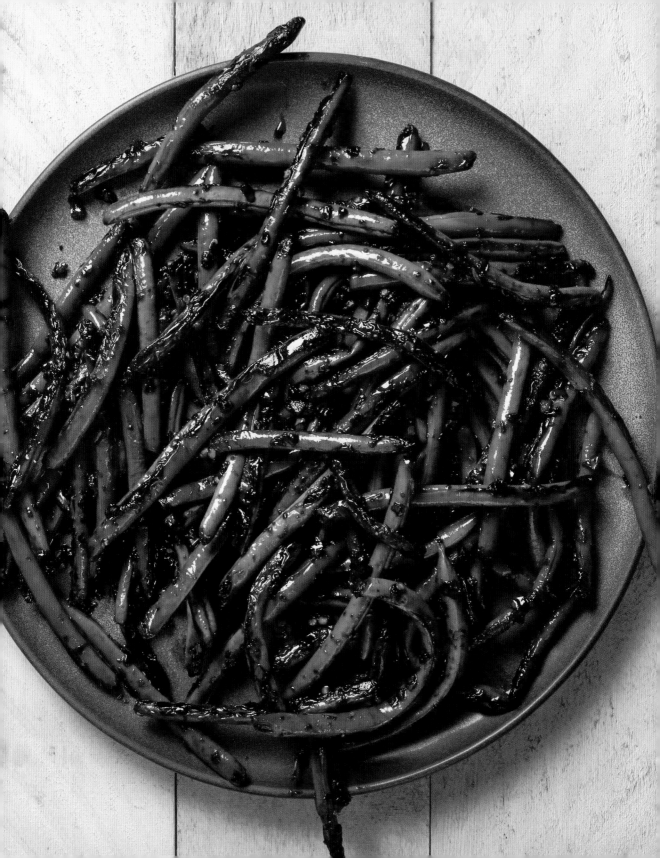

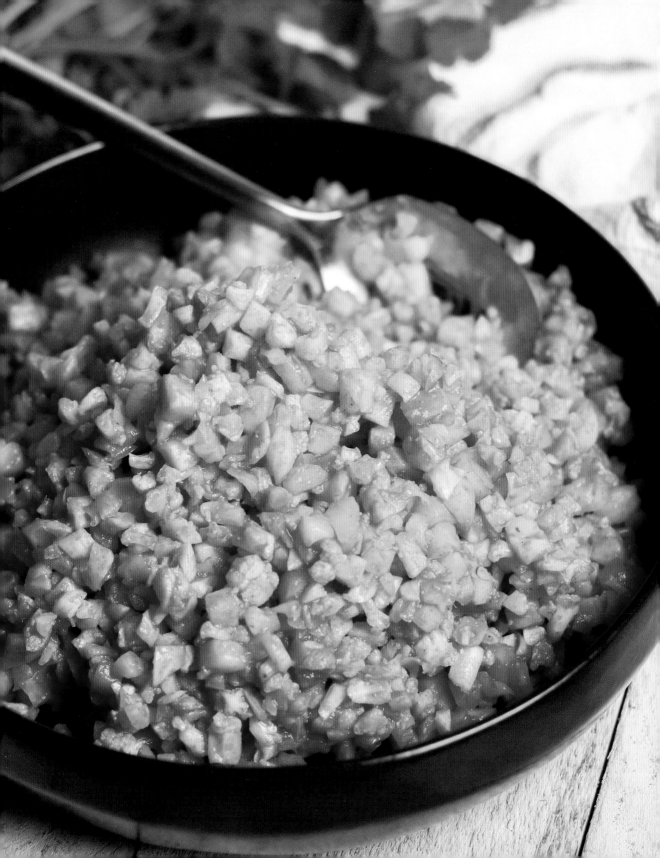

ab 5-minute spanish rice

you follow me on Instagram, you probably already know that I do not normally like auliflower rice because it's often soggy and watery. But not here! Here, we do it right. ne trick is twofold: One, using fresh cauliflower rice, not frozen. Two, not overcooking . This version is inspired by the Mexican-style *arroz rojo*—often called Spanish rice in ne U.S. It's seasoned with tomato, spices and bouillon to give it its signature flavor and lowing red color. And it really works as a perfect side to basically any meat or seafood ish, although it lends itself particularly well to Tex-Mex and Mexican cuisine, of course. nd even for me, a true cauli-rice dissenter, I absolutely love it!

y pairing this with the Austin Food Truck Breakfast Tacos (for Dinner!) on page 65.

tbsp (30 ml) avocado oil

tbsp (14 g) unsalted butter (optional)

(14-oz [397-g]) bags fresh riced cauliflower ot frozen)

(8-oz [226-g]) can tomato sauce

1 tbsp (7 g) chicken bouillon powder

1 tsp garlic powder

1 tsp cumin

2 tsp (4 g) sweet paprika

Varm a large (12-inch [30-cm]) skillet over medium-high heat. Once it's hot, add the avocado oil nd butter to the pan. As the butter starts to melt, add the cauliflower, tomato sauce, chicken bouillon, arlic powder, cumin and paprika, and stir really well. Sauté for 2 minutes, stirring continuously. Turn f the heat and immediately pour the rice into a serving bowl—remember, the trick with this recipe is ot overcooking the cauliflower. When you turn off the heat, the cauliflower should still have a little bite it (al dente) because it will continue cooking after you take it off the heat. It's best to serve this right way, so I suggest making this dish just as dinner is about to be served.

pro tip: This quick recipe is a very simple side dish to go with any meal. But to make it the star of the show, dress it up by adding sautéed peppers, onions, jalapeños or even meat, like chorizo or seasoned ground beef.

---

serves
6

active cooking time
5 minutes

total time
5 minutes

---

macros per serving

calories
106

protein
4.3 g

fat
6.7 g

net carbs
5.5 g

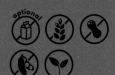

serves
4

**active cooking
time**
20 minutes

total time
20 minutes

**macros per
serving**

calories
232

protein
4.3 g

fat
23.1 g

net carbs
2.2 g

herby pan-roasted mushrooms

Butter, herbs and mushrooms: a trio sent from heaven! Sure, it sounds simple, but something magical happens when the mushrooms soak up all that deliciousness. You just have to try it to find out for yourself. Serve these with steak or chicken, or here just eat the whole pan of it yourself. Either way, you won't regret it. Shhh, I won't tell anyone if you top these with some Parmesan cheese too. In fact, I encourage it.

Try pairing this with the Blue Cheese Lovers' Steak and Asparagus Sauté on page 33.

1 lb (454 g) whole baby bella (or cremini) mushrooms

½ cup (114 g) unsalted butter (see Pro Tip)

½ tsp sea salt

½ tsp freshly cracked black pepper

½ tsp garlic powder

½ tsp herbes de Provence

½ tbsp (2 g) chopped packed fresh parsley

Preheat the oven to 375°F (190°C) and use a damp paper towel to wipe any dirt off the mushroom

Place a large (12-inch [30-cm]) oven-safe skillet over medium heat and add the butter. Once the butter is fully melted, add the mushrooms, salt, black pepper, garlic powder and herbes de Provence. Sauté for 2 minutes, or until the butter gets brown and fragrant. Place the skillet in the oven for 10 minutes, until the mushrooms are fork tender. Sprinkle the chopped parsley on top of the mushrooms and enjoy

pro tip: For a dairy-free, vegan and lower-calorie version, swap the butter with olive oil.

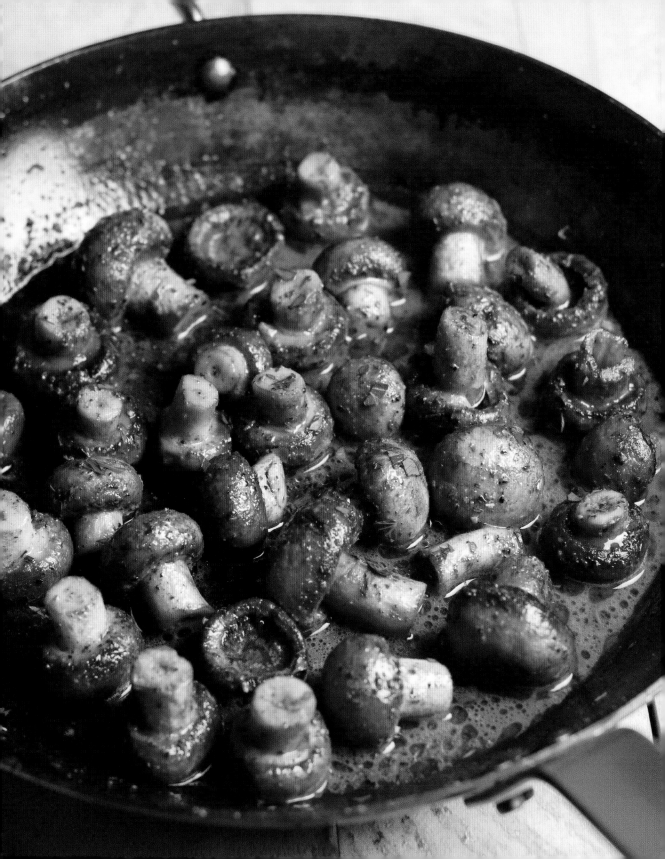

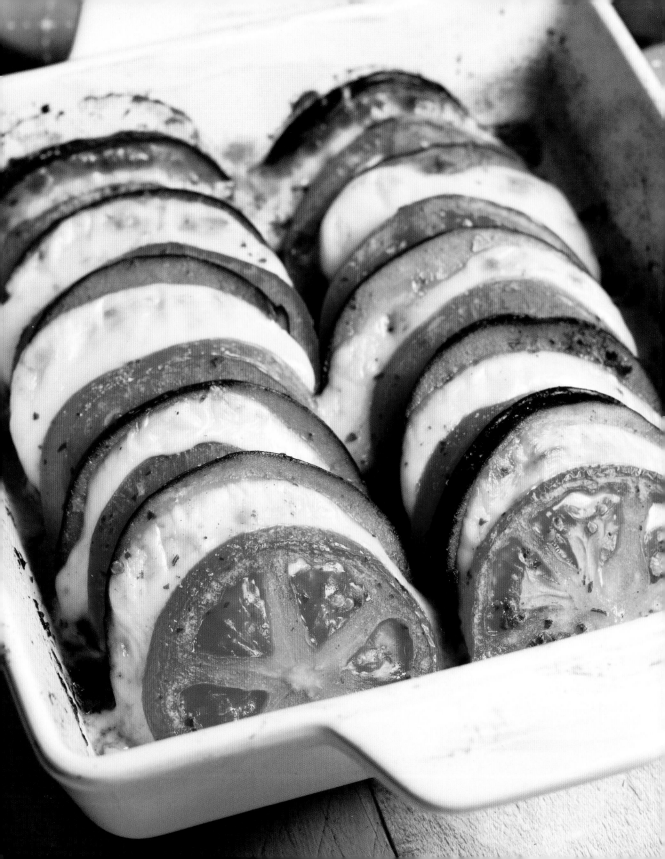

beautifully layered eggplant caprese

This gorgeous side dish speaks for itself. Layers of meaty eggplant, juicy tomatoes and melty mozzarella come together perfectly in this stunning side dish. And the pesto infusion adds a beautiful, herbaceous flavor to the veggies. If you don't love eggplant, use zucchini instead. If you have any leftover vegetables from this recipe, don't throw them away! Chop them up and use them in the Lemony Spice-Roasted Mixed Veggies on page 130.

Try pairing this with the Parmesan-Crusted Chicken Piccata on page 57.

small eggplant (15 oz [425 g] or less)

large beefsteak or salad tomatoes

½ cup (120 g) basil pesto (from a jar)

2 tbsp (30 ml) extra virgin olive oil

1 tbsp (15 ml) balsamic vinegar

¼ tsp + ⅛ tsp sea salt, divided

1 (8-oz [226-g]) ball fresh mozzarella, pre-sliced in the package or thinly sliced

Preheat the oven to 475°F (240°C).

Cut off the stem ends of the eggplant and tomatoes, and then thinly slice them into ¼-inch (6-mm) rounds (see Pro Tip). In total, you'll need 10 slices of each. Place the eggplant slices into a 9 x 9–inch (23 x 23–cm) baking dish, and then add on top of the eggplant the pesto, olive oil, balsamic and ¼ teaspoon of salt. Use your hands to massage the mixture all over the sliced eggplant, covering all sides evenly. Then, arrange the vegetables in two rows by layering the tomato and mozzarella between the eggplant slices (almost like roof shingles). Sprinkle the top of the veggies evenly with the remaining salt, and place the dish into the oven to bake for 20 to 25 minutes, or until the eggplant is fork-tender. Switch the oven to broil and cook for 2 minutes, or just until the cheese gets lightly browned and bubbly. Take the dish out of the oven and serve family-style.

pro tip: Did you know that the best way to cut a tomato is using a serrated bread knife? It helps prevent the tomato from getting squished while slicing.

serves
4

active cooking time
10 minutes

total time
30 minutes

macros per serving

calories
329

protein
14.9 g

fat
24.8 g

net carbs
6.2 g

serves
6

active cooking time
10 minutes

total time
30 minutes

macros per serving

calories
126

protein
3.6 g

fat
9.5 g

net carbs
6.8 g

lemony spice-roasted mixed veggies

Sometimes simple is better, and this is one of those times. But these simply roasted vegetables are anything but boring. They are coated in a stunning blend of spices with a Mediterranean flair, so these veggies are exploding with flavor. Don't be discouraged by the long list of ingredients—those are mostly spices, which you almost certainly already have in your pantry. Packed with healthy vitamins and nutrients, this easy sheet-pan side dish is simply beautiful and pairs perfectly with almost any dinner you can imagine.

Try pairing this with the Succulent Spanish Garlic Shrimp (Gambas al Ajillo) on page 90

1 zucchini, cut into half-moons

1 summer (yellow) squash, cut into half-moons

6 oz (170 g) broccolini or broccoli, stems trimmed

8 oz (226 g) baby bella (cremini) mushrooms, sliced in half

10 oz (283 g) grape tomatoes

8 cloves garlic

¼ cup (60 ml) fresh lemon juice (from 2 lemons)

¼ cup (60 ml) extra virgin olive oil

1 tsp sea salt

1 tsp freshly cracked black pepper

2 tsp (4 g) garlic powder

1 tsp onion powder

1 tsp cumin

2 tsp (2 g) dried dill

¼ tsp cinnamon

2 tsp (4 g) sweet paprika

Preheat the oven to 475°F (240°C) and line a baking sheet with parchment paper or aluminum foil.

In a large bowl, add the zucchini, squash, broccolini, mushrooms, tomatoes, garlic, lemon juice, olive oil, salt, black pepper, garlic powder, onion powder, cumin, dill, cinnamon and paprika. Toss with your hands until the veggies are evenly coated in the spices. Pour everything out onto the lined baking sheet and spread in an even layer. Bake for 20 minutes, or until the veggies are soft and lightly browned. Serve this family-style or onto individual plates.

pro tip: This is a great recipe to use up any leftover veggies you have in the fridge. So, feel free to swap in any of your favorite veggies that might be heading toward their expiration date. For example, asparagus, red onion, butternut squash or cauliflower would all be really delicious in this dish.

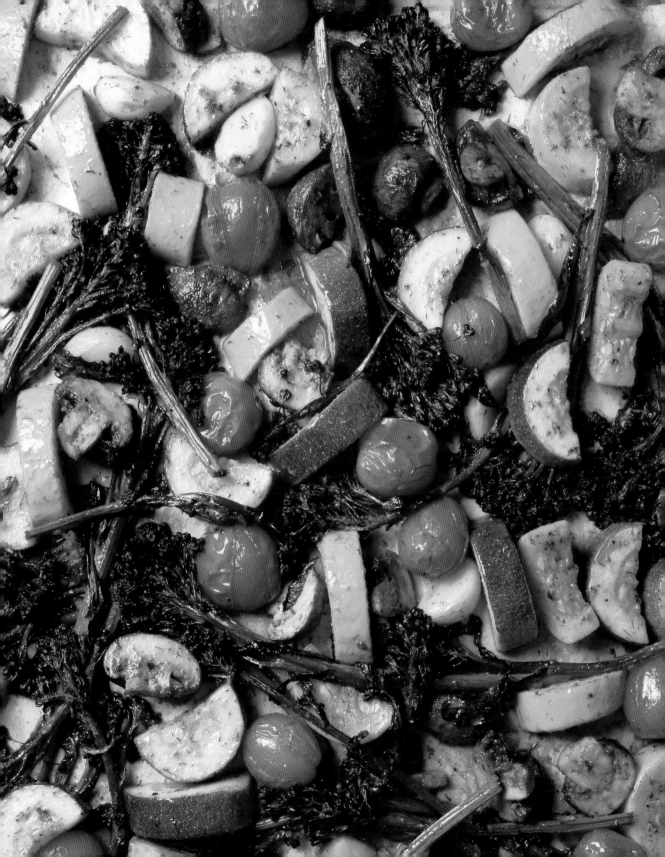

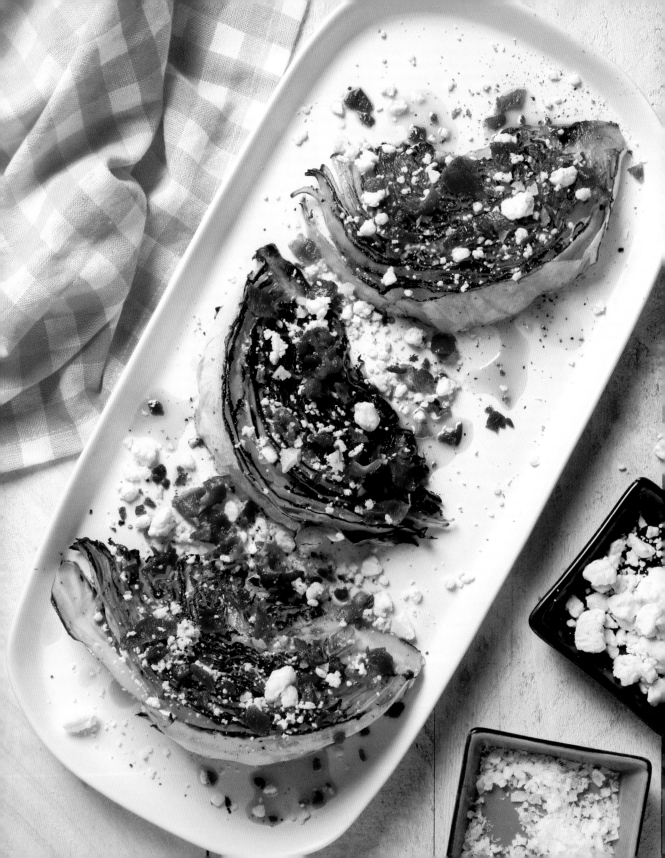

Fabulous bacon-fried cabbage steaks

Roll out the red carpet! Cabbage finally had its glow up! This recipe takes the humblest vegetable and turns it into a showstopping hero. The cabbage "steaks" are fried to perfection, then covered in salty bacon, creamy goat cheese and a squeeze of lemon. So don't believe what they say about you, cabbage . . . you are so much more than just slaw. Everyone deserves their chance to shine, so cabbage, this is your moment!

Try pairing this with the Firecracker Chicken Meatballs on page 41.

serves
4

active cooking time
25 minutes

total time
25 minutes

macros per serving

calories
195

protein
7.9 g

fat
16 g

net carbs
4.9 g

---

head green cabbage, halved

tbsp (15 ml) avocado oil

¼ tsp sea salt

oz (170 g) no-sugar bacon

½ cup (120 ml) chicken broth

2 tbsp (30 ml) extra virgin olive oil

1 tbsp (15 ml) fresh lemon juice (from ½ lemon)

2 tbsp (19 g) crumbled goat cheese (optional; see Pro Tip)

¼ tsp freshly cracked black pepper

Flaky finishing salt, chopped parsley and sliced scallions, to serve (optional)

Remove the outer two leaves from the cabbage. Leaving the stem on, cut the cabbage in half, stem to tip. *Note: This recipe only uses half a cabbage, so wrap up the other half in plastic wrap and save it in your fridge.* Cut the cabbage half into four equal-sized wedges (steaks), ensuring that you leave a little bit of the stem attached to every wedge. (This will prevent the cabbage from falling apart in the pan.) Rub the cabbage steaks with the avocado oil and sea salt on both sides. Set them aside.

Place a large (12-inch [30-cm]) cast-iron skillet on the stove and line it with the bacon. Turn on the heat to medium, and cook the bacon for 8 minutes, or until it's crispy, flipping it halfway through. Take the bacon out of the pan and set it aside on a plate. Leaving the bacon fat in the pan, turn the heat up to medium-high, and pour in the chicken broth. Use a spatula to stir the bottom of the pan to remove the fond (the browned bits stuck to the bottom of the pan). Place the four cabbage steaks into the pan, and cook for 6 minutes, or until all the liquid in the pan has evaporated and the steaks have a nice dark-brown sear. Very carefully flip over each steak with a spatula and let them cook for 4 minutes on the other side.

Chop the bacon into small pieces. Take the cabbage wedges out of the pan and plate them on a serving platter. Drizzle them with the olive oil and lemon juice. Sprinkle the tops with the crumbled goat cheese (if using), chopped bacon and black pepper. Garnish with flaky salt, parsley or scallions (if using).

pro tip: Don't like goat cheese? Feta, blue cheese or Parmesan also work great! Or just leave it out for a dairy-free version.

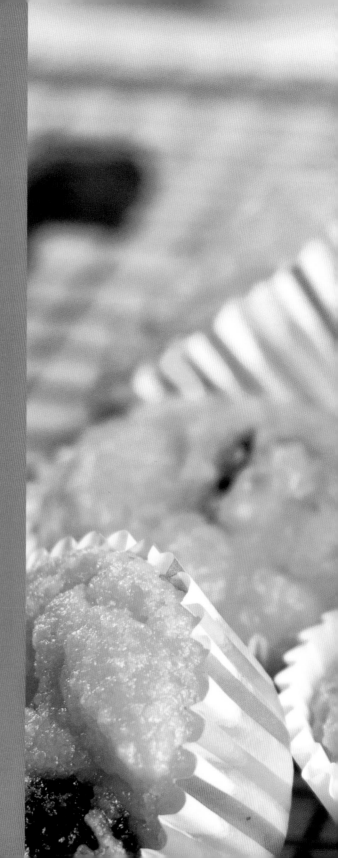

swift sweets

You know when you're sitting on the couch after dinner, and suddenly it hits you? The I-just-need-a-little-something-sweet alarm goes off in your head. Well, that's exactly what these recipes are—small and healthy sweet bites you can make in a hurry. They may not feed a crowd, but who said you were sharing, anyway?

Boozy Margarita Mug Cake (page 136)

Seductive Strawberry Mojito Fool (page 139)

Blueberry Lemon Mini Muffins (page 140)

Chewy Ginger Almond Butter Cookies (page 143)

Mike's Midnight Munchie Bars (page 144)

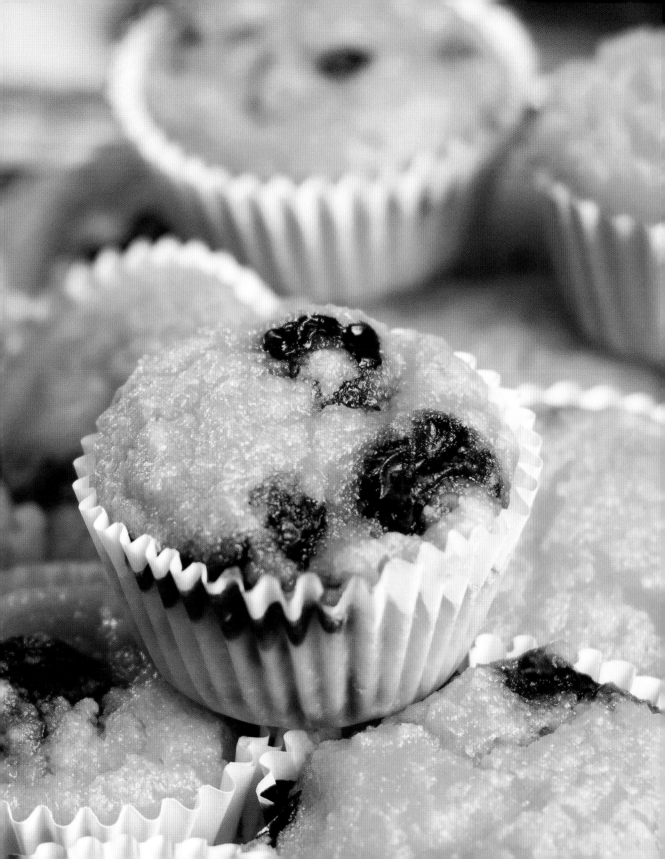

makes
1 mug cake

active cooking time
15 minutes

total time
15 minutes

macros per serving

calories
313

protein
7.7 g

fat
24.5 g

net carbs
3.8 g

boozy margarita mug cake

It's five o'clock somewhere, isn't it? Either way, this fiesta-worthy mug cake is as tasty a it is cute. And let's not forget, it's flourless and sugar-free, so you can have one of these anytime you want. Of course, the tequila is optional, since these little cakes are just a delicious without it. The zesty lime flavor is tangy and refreshing, and the sweet glaze or top balances it all out. So, booze or no booze, it's happy hour with this recipe!

vanilla lime mug cake

1 egg

3 tbsp (21 g) almond flour

1 tbsp (14 g) granulated sweetener (I recommend allulose)

½ tsp vanilla extract

½ tsp baking powder

Zest from 1 lime

½ tbsp (8 ml) fresh lime juice (from ½ lime)

1 tbsp (14 g) unsalted butter

tequila-lime glaze

1 tbsp (8 g) sifted confectioners sweetener

1 tsp tequila or fresh lime juice

Chili-lime seasoning or kosher salt and lime slices, to serve (optional)

To make the mug cake, in a small bowl, beat the egg well with a fork. Add the almond flour, sweetener vanilla, baking powder, zest and lime juice. Mix well to combine, and then set the bowl aside. In c coffee mug, add the butter, and microwave it for 60 seconds to melt it completely. Roll the butter arounc in the mug to coat all the walls—get as close to the top of the mug as possible. Pour the remaining butter that's in the mug into the bowl with the batter, and stir until combined. Pour the batter into the mug Place the mug in the microwave, and cook on high for 60 seconds. Set it aside to cool.

To make the glaze, in a small bowl, mix together the confectioners sweetener and tequila and whisk Drizzle the glaze over the top of the mug cake. Garnish your "margarita" with the chili-lime seasoning or salt and lime slices (if using).

pro tips: For a fun upgrade, mince a strawberry and stir it into the mug cake batter before cooking it. Then add a sliced strawberry on top of the finished cake for a Strawberry Lime version. And to really dress up this little treat, try topping it with a dollop of homemade whipped cream.

If you don't love lime, try it with lemon or orange instead!

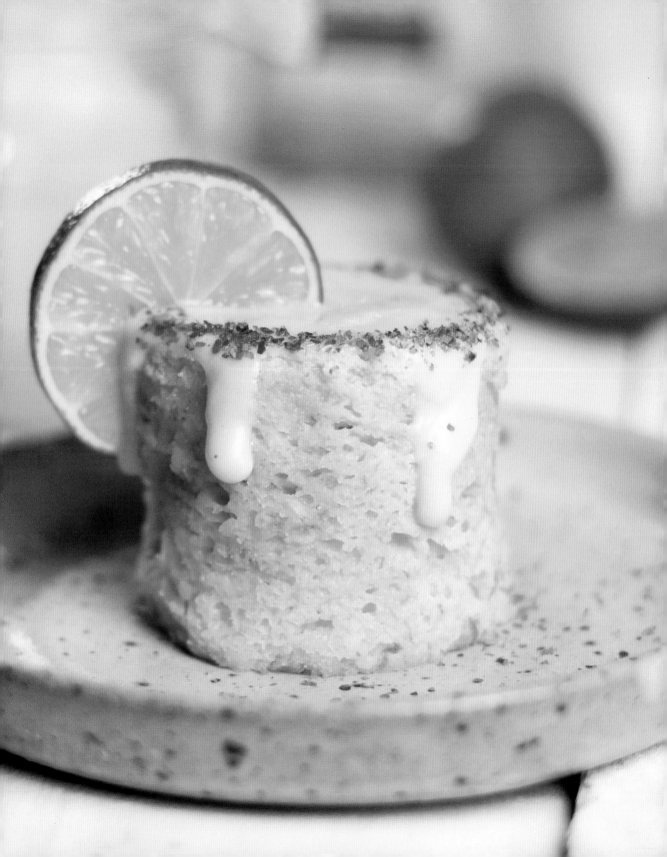

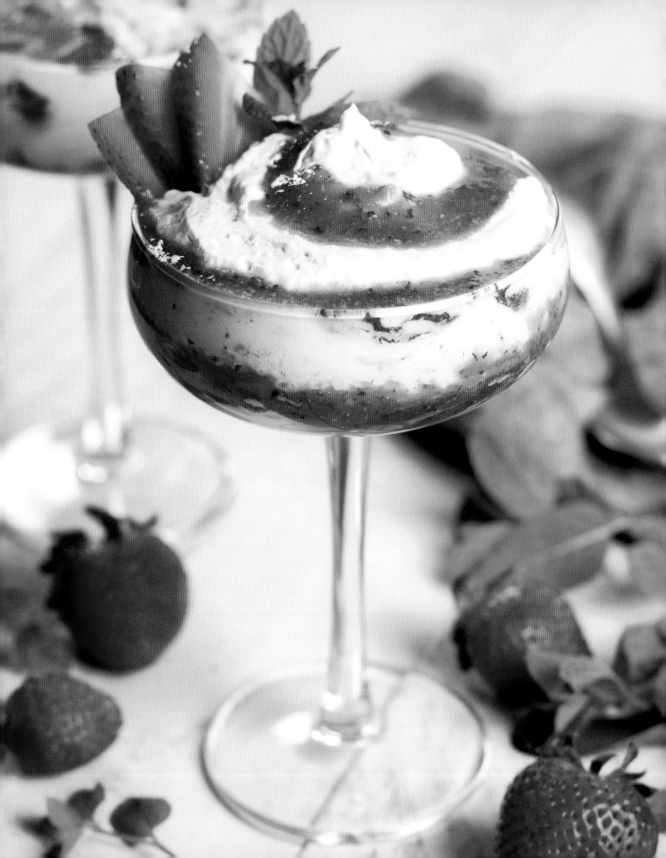

seductive strawberry mojito fool

here's only one fool around here . . . and that's you if you don't make this tasty treat!
m kidding, obviously. A "fool" is a British dessert that combines fruit puree with custard
r whipped cream. So because this is an English recipe, I suppose I'll dedicate this to the
an who's called me a fool many times over. This one's for you, Gordon Ramsay. To
y mentor, my inspiration and the greatest chef I've ever known, thank you for seeing
omething in me that I never even saw in myself.

oz (226 g) fresh strawberries, plus extra for
arnish

tbsp (6 g) roughly chopped packed fresh mint
aves, stems removed, plus extra for garnish

2 cup (108 g) granulated sweetener
recommend allulose)

½ tbsp (8 ml) fresh lime juice (from ½ lime)

1 cup (240 ml) heavy cream

1 tsp vanilla extract

ut the stems off the strawberries, and slice the berries in half. Add them to a food processor with the
int, sweetener and lime juice. Blend on high for 1 minute, or until the mixture gets smooth.

a medium bowl, add the heavy cream and vanilla, and use a hand or standing mixer to whip the
ream on high for 2 to 3 minutes, or until it forms stiff peaks. Pour half of the strawberry puree into
he bowl and whip for 1 minute, or until it forms stiff peaks again. Layer in the whipped cream with the
emaining strawberry puree in small glasses or bowls. Top with strawberry slices and mint leaves. Serve
ght away or store them in the fridge, covered, for up to 3 days.

pro tip: This is equally delicious using raspberries instead of strawberries. You can
also shave some sugar-free dark chocolate on top for a decadent upgrade.

serves
4

**active cooking
time**
20 minutes

total time
20 minutes

**macros per
serving**

calories
230

protein
1.8 g

fat
22.2 g

net carbs
5.3 g

makes
20 mini muffins

active cooking time
10 minutes

total time
30 minutes

macros per muffin

calories
52

protein
1.7 g

fat
3.6 g

net carbs
1.6 g

blueberry lemon mini muffins

Kid friendly, parent approved! These little bites remind me of the mini muffins I had a a kid, but much, much better. And they are Keto-friendly and sugar-free, so they real are perfect little sweets. The blueberries burst with juicy flavor, and the lemon give them a subtle tang and golden color. So whether you're making these for the kids or fo yourself, you'll wish you made a double batch.

1 cup (122 g) almond flour

1 tbsp (7 g) coconut flour

1 tsp baking powder

⅛ tsp sea salt

1 cup (216 g) granulated sweetener (I recommend allulose)

Zest from 1 lemon

2 eggs

¼ cup (60 ml) sour cream

1 tbsp (15 ml) fresh lemon juice (from ½ lemon)

1 tsp vanilla extract

1 cup (148 g) blueberries

Preheat the oven to 350°F (180°C) and line a mini muffin tin with paper liners.

In a large bowl, combine the almond flour, coconut flour, baking powder, salt, sweetener and lemo zest. Whisk to remove any lumps. Add the eggs, sour cream, lemon juice and vanilla, and mix until th batter is smooth. Stir in the blueberries. With a spoon, divide the mixture evenly into the mini muffin tir (I used about 1 tablespoon [15 ml] of batter per muffin.) Fill the cups just shy of the top of the liner t allow the muffin to expand. Bake for 20 minutes. Take the pan out of the oven and set it aside to coo Once cooled, remove the muffins from the tin, and enjoy!

pro tip: These keep well in the freezer, so you can make a big batch and store them in an airtight container or bag in the freezer. Pop them in the toaster oven to warm them up whenever you need a quick sweet treat or an on-the-go breakfast.

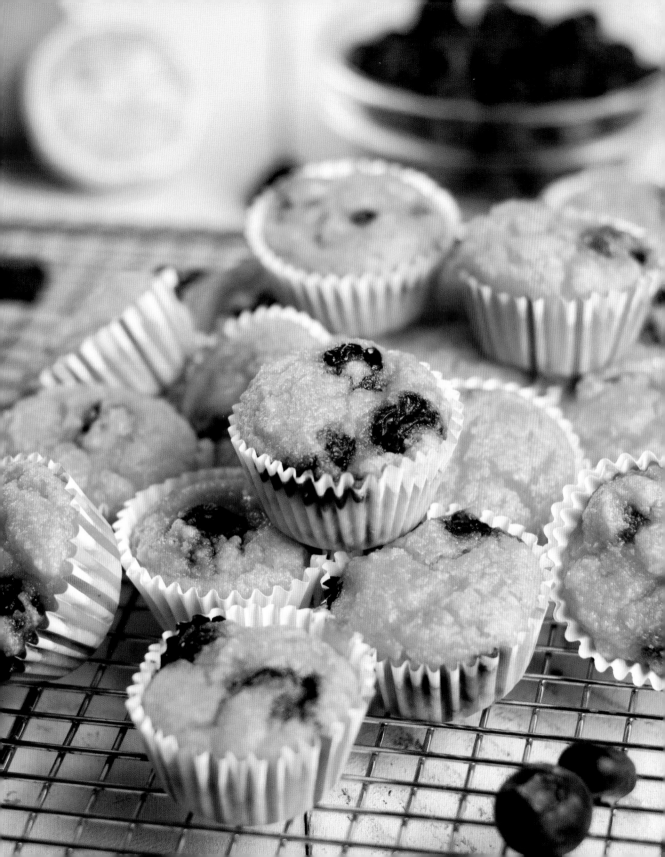

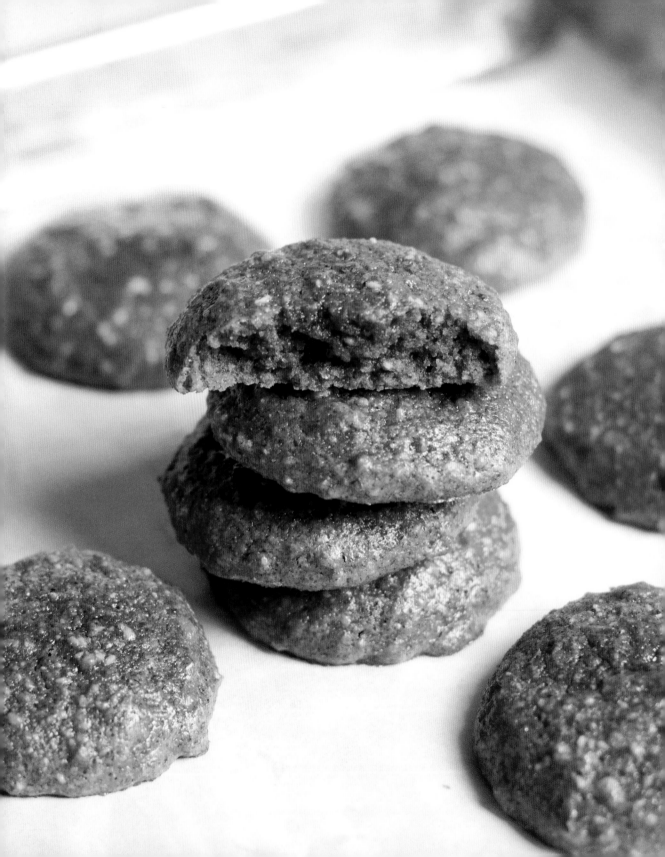

chewy ginger almond butter cookies

These little cookies are gooey, chewy and oh, so delicious. They remind me of gingersnap cookies with their warm, wintry spices. But they're really a protein-packed, on-the-go snack for the whole family, thanks to the almond butter base. They are flourless, sugar-free, guilt-free cookies, so you can have as many as you'd like. And they're great for the holidays too.

cup (129 g) almond butter

tsp vanilla extract

egg

pinch of sea salt

cup (72 g) granulated sweetener
recommend allulose)

1 tbsp (8 g) cinnamon

1½ tbsp (8 g) ground ginger

½ tsp ground clove

Preheat the oven to 350°F (180°C).

In a large bowl, add the almond butter, vanilla, egg, salt, sweetener, cinnamon, ginger and clove. Mix until the batter is evenly combined. Use a spoon (see Pro Tip) to scoop the mixture (2 tablespoons [30 ml] per cookie) onto a baking sheet, 1 inch (2.5 cm) apart. If you wet your fingers with a little water, you can mold and shape the cookies to be even and round. Bake for 10 minutes, or just until the cookies are glossy and set. Remove the pan from the oven and set aside to let the cookies cool for 5 minutes before taking them off the pan. Let them cool completely before serving or storing in an airtight container in the fridge for up to 3 days. You can also make them ahead of time and freeze them until you're ready to serve.

pro tip: For perfectly round and even cookies, muffins or cupcakes, get a set of ice cream scoops. I suggest getting a three-pack that comes with different sizes. It really helps when baking, and they really do come in handy, especially if you bake a lot. For this recipe, you can use a small ice cream scoop.

makes
10 small cookies

active cooking time
15 minutes

total time
25 minutes

macros per cookie

calories
92

protein
2.3 g

fat
7.9 g

net carbs
2.5 g

makes
8 small or 4 large candy bars

active cooking time
15 minutes

total time
30 minutes

macros per serving

calories
237

protein
1.6 g

fat
25.5 g

net carbs
3.2 g

mike's midnight munchie bars

We've all been there. That late-night craving for something sweet hits. Instead of reaching for that naughty chocolate bar, why not make your own instead? This recipe is fun and highly customizable. And don't be intimidated by the long list of instructions below; this is super easy to make. You basically melt chocolate and mix it with your favorite nuts or mix-ins. This is just my favorite combination: dark chocolate, flaky salt, crunchy macadamia nuts and crispy coconut. But you make it however you'd like! Try hazelnuts, peanuts, pistachios or even dried fruit. Try it with milk or white chocolate. No matter what, your midnight munchies now have a perfectly craveable and guilt-free solution.

1 cup (146 g) macadamia nuts

7 oz (198 g) sugar-free dark chocolate chips (I recommend ChocZero® or Lily's® brand)

1 tbsp (14 g) coconut oil

½ cup (50 g) unsweetened coconut flakes

¼ tsp flaky finishing salt or sea salt

Add the macadamia nuts to a sandwich-sized ziplock bag. Seal the bag tightly, removing the air, and use the bottom of a pan or a rolling pin to crack them into slightly smaller pieces. Set the bag aside. Fill a small saucepan with just enough water to cover the bottom, and place it over high heat. Grab a heat-safe bowl and set it on top of the pot on the stove, making a "double boiler." Once the water is boiling, lower the heat to medium-low, and add the chocolate chips and coconut oil to the bowl on top. Use a spatula to continuously stir the chocolate until the chips are 90 percent melted (a few small lumps are okay). Turn off the heat. This process should only take 1 to 2 minutes. Slide the double boiler, including the pot, off the burner, but leave the chocolate bowl sitting on top to stay warm.

Warm a large (12-inch [30-cm]) skillet over medium-high heat. Once hot, add the crushed macadamia nuts and coconut flakes. Toast the nuts in the pan, stirring constantly for 2 to 3 minutes, or until the coconut just starts to turn golden brown. Don't walk away from the pan, as these can burn very quickly. Immediately pour the nuts onto a plate to stop the cooking process. Set aside about ½ cup (75 g) of the toasted mixture to use later for topping. Pour the rest of the mixture into the bowl of chocolate and stir together well.

Using a silicone candy bar mold, fill up the wells of the mold evenly with the chocolate mixture. Sprinkle the bars with the flaky salt and top with the remaining coconut and macadamia mixture. Place the bars into the freezer for 15 minutes to cool and set. Store them in a sealed bag in the fridge or pantry, and pop one out whenever you're ready for a munchie!

pro tip: For an even easier version, turn these into chocolate "bark" instead! Skip the silicone molds and simply pour the chocolate mixture onto a parchment-lined baking sheet, then add the toppings. Once cool and firm, break the chocolate into pieces.

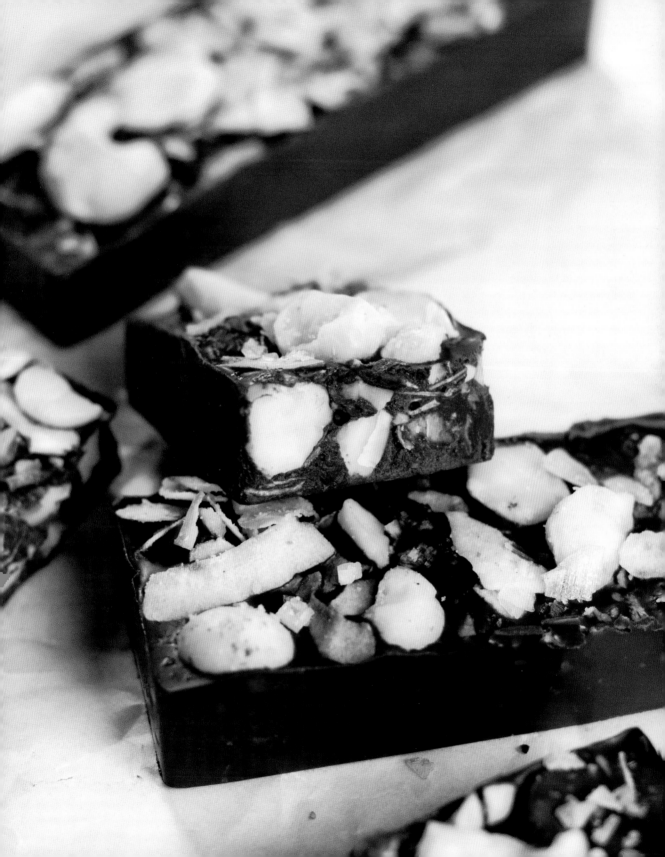

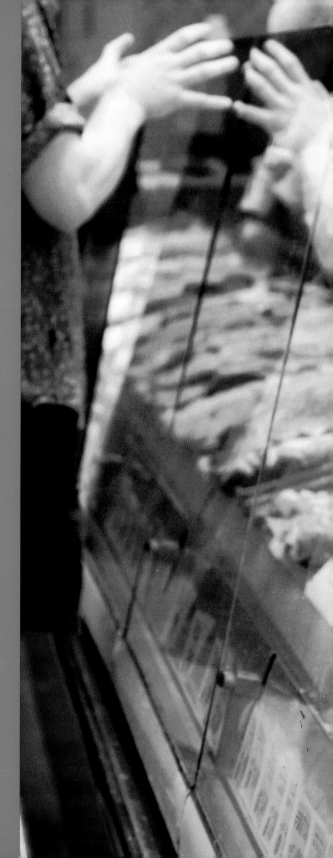

chef's cheat sheet

What kind of knife should I use? Which cut of steak should I buy? How do I know if this chicken is cooked? I got you covered! Think of this chapter as your personal cheat sheet for the kitchen. Full of tips and information, this section will help you get perfect results every time, from the grocery store right down to your serving plate.

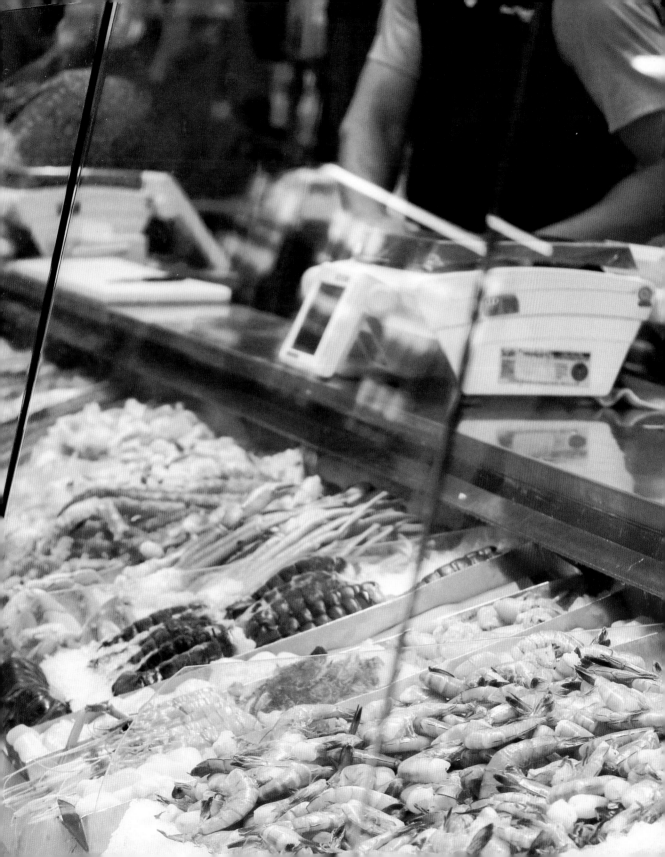

tips and tricks: saving time and money

I get it—most nights, we just need to get food on the table. And this book is filled with great recipes to do just that. But in this section, I also wanted to give you a few extra ideas to help you cook my recipes even quicker, and to save a few bucks along the way.

Time-Saving Tips

Shopping for Speed

If you're in a hurry, wandering the aisles of the grocery store is not the answer. Make a shopping list ahead of time, and stick to it. Better yet, take advantage of curbside pickup! If you planned your menu for the week, shop for it online, order it ahead and let someone else do the shopping. And don't be afraid to buy pre-sliced veggies. Slicing those onions or trimming those green beans could add 5 to 10 minutes to your prep time that you might not have. Just keep in mind, sometimes precut veggies cost a bit more, so it won't help your budget. But time is money, right?

Doubling Down

Almost every recipe in this book can easily be doubled or tripled. When I cook, I almost always make double, because the leftovers inevitably become tomorrow's lunch or dinner. This can also be really helpful for meal prepping, so you can pack lunches for work. Bringing lunch to work can really save you money and keep you away from the temptations of fast food and office donuts.

Implementing Mise en Place

Mise en place, borrowed from the French phrase for "everything in place," is the chef's term for all your "prep work." It's really the key to moving quickly and efficiently in the kitchen. So, before you start cooking, or even grocery shopping, read the recipe all the way through. Take note of the prep instructions in the ingredient list, such as "chopped" or "thinly sliced." Get out any equipment you'll need, and precut and measure all your ingredients. This will ensure the recipe goes as smooth as butter.

Working Like a Chef

Work smarter, not harder—keep your kitchen organized and clean as you go. This will allow you to focus on the tasks in front of you. And if you clean a little as you go, when dinner's over, you won't have a pile of dishes to conquer. Put away ingredients as you use them, wipe down your counters and rinse off the dishes before the contents dry on the plate.

Staying Stocked

The best way to ensure you stick to your dinner plans at home is to set yourself up for success. Plan out your meals, shop only once a week and keep your pantry and fridge full of the basic items you need at all times—things such as ground beef, chicken, frozen shrimp, herbs, spices and basic veggies— and you can easily throw a few of your favorite recipes together without much planning. See the Pantry Principles on page 150 for more ideas for keeping your kitchen well stocked.

Bang for Your Buck

Buying in Bulk

This one may seem obvious, but hear me out. Clearly, buying in bulk will get you more food per dollar. And in most cases, this is a great way to save money. But there is a caveat to this: buying more than you really need. Warehouse stores are a fantastic way to stock up on your most-needed items—especially if you have a big family to feed. But there are times where it doesn't make sense, especially with perishable goods that can go bad before you use them. So focus on buying only the bulk items you know you need, and shop for the rest at your local supermarket. Also, start using the unit prices when comparing products, rather than the total cost or size of the box.

Supermarket Sweep

Do not underestimate the money-saving power of shopping at a discount grocery store. There are many discount grocery stores or even grocery outlets around the U.S. and abroad that can help you save big bucks. I also highly recommend you shop at your local international markets as well. You can find amazing prices on fresh produce, spices and meat/seafood at Latin, Asian or Indian grocery stores.

Wasted Wages

We all shop with the intention of eating all those fresh veggies, but sadly, many just don't make it into our meals and inevitably end up getting thrown away. So planning your meals ahead so you only shop for what you need is key. Properly storing fruits and vegetables in sealed containers and keeping an eye on the expiration dates on the meat and dairy are critical to preventing wasted dollars.

Freezer Frenzy

Freeze what you won't use! Whether it's the extra meat in the package you've bought in bulk, or your leftovers, don't let them go to waste! I suggest freezing extra meat in individual portions so you can more easily thaw them for future recipes. If you have any fruits or veggies approaching their expiration, cut them up and freeze them in ziplock bags to use later in soups and stews. Freeze your fruit in bags to use later in smoothies. And before you put your food in the freezer, use a permanent marker to label the bag with its contents and the date, so later you know what it is, and when you froze it.

Only the Outer Aisle

The first time I heard this concept, I had to pause to think about it. But it's profoundly simple: Stay away from the central, snack food aisles, and focus on the perimeter of the supermarket. That's where you find produce, meat, seafood, deli and dairy. Not only will this help you buy healthier, meal-focused ingredients rather than snacks, but it'll help keep you away from all the tempting (and expensive!) junk foods. Other than a few canned goods and spices, almost every recipe in this book can be made primarily using only the outer aisle of the grocery store.

More Money-Saving Moves

- Buy generic! Most generic products are of equal quality to the name brands. In fact, many are even made in the same factories.

- You don't need to buy fancy, organic health foods all the time—just do the best you can based on your own budget. If you're focusing on food quality, aim for locally sourced foods and shop at the local farmers' market for the best quality at the lowest prices.

- Shop online, especially for low-carb/dietary ingredients. The specialty foods get really expensive at the grocery store, so ordering your Keto basics online can definitely lighten the load.

- Use a grocery app like Fetch or Ibotta for digital coupons and rebates on the food you buy. These apps are free, and the savings add up.

pantry principles

Buying the Basics

Throughout this book, you'll notice that many of the recipes use certain ingredients over and over. That is not an accident. I want you to be able to shop for one recipe, but secretly get two or three more dinners out of it. Below, I've created a basic pantry list that you can use to stock your kitchen. These ingredients will be universal enough to use again and again. And instead of shopping for a million ingredients every week, you can focus on quickly grabbing just a few fresh veggies and proteins that you can get several meals out of, knowing that at home you have all the other pantry essentials ready to go. Keep these essentials in stock, and you'll be cooking like a pro!

Spices and Seasonings

- Adobo or seasoning salt
- Black pepper
- Cajun seasoning or Old Bay
- Chili powder
- Cinnamon
- Crushed red pepper flakes
- Cumin
- Dried dill
- Dried Italian herb blend
- Dried oregano
- Garlic powder
- Ground ginger
- Onion powder
- Sea salt
- Sweet and Smoked Paprika

Condiments and Oils

- Apple cider vinegar
- Avocado oil
- Balsamic vinegar
- Chicken and beef bouillon powder
- Dijon mustard
- Extra virgin olive oil
- Mayonnaise
- Nonstick cooking spray
- No-sugar barbecue sauce
- No-sugar ketchup
- Salted and unsalted butter
- Sesame oil
- Soy sauce (or coconut aminos)
- Worcestershire sauce

Cans, Jars and Dry Goods

- Canned tomato sauce
- Chipotle peppers in adobo
- Coconut cream (unsweetened)
- Fire-roasted tomatoes and green chilies
- Low-carb pasta/rice
- Low-carb tortillas
- No-sugar marinara
- Sun-dried tomatoes (in oil)
- Tomato paste

Sugar Showdown

To sugar or not to sugar? Well, that is the question. And there is no universal answer. If you're looking to remove sugars and carbs from your diet, using sugar alternatives (sweeteners) may be very helpful.

So which sweetener is right for you? It's a very personal decision, and you'll have to do a little self-experimentation to find out which sweetener is best for your body and lifestyle. You may find that a given sweetener gives you a stomachache or leaves a bad aftertaste, but that will differ vastly from person to person. Here are the four sweeteners I'd recommend you use; they all have a low glycemic impact (the effect on blood glucose and insulin levels) and are considered safe to use.

Allulose

Allulose is a newer, low-calorie sugar substitute on the market, and it's called a rare sugar because it's found only in small quantities in nature (in fruits like figs and raisins). It's my personal favorite because it cooks and caramelizes the most like real sugar. It has a great taste and almost no aftertaste or cooling effect. But it's still generally harder to find than the other sweeteners, although it's starting to pop up in more and more regular supermarkets. I order mine online for the best pricing. *Note: It is not yet available in Canada or Europe.*

Erythritol

A sugar-alcohol, found in products like Swerve, erythritol is a good sugar-free option, and works well in baking, but it leaves many people with a "cooling" aftertaste and tends to crystallize in sauces and in liquids. Note: It will not properly caramelize, so be careful with this one in sauces and caramels.

Monk Fruit

This is another great option, but monk fruit is often blended with other sweeteners, so read the product labels. It can have a strong aftertaste for many people as well, but it's a good natural option.

Stevia

Naturally derived from the stevia leaf, stevia sweeteners, especially liquid stevia, can be around 100 times sweeter than sugar, so use it sparingly. Read the label to find the correct sugar conversion rate. You may only need a tiny bit of it in a recipe to get the desired sweetness. *Note: For some, stevia has a strong aftertaste, but try it for yourself.*

Sweeteners to Avoid

Stay away from maltitol, maltodextrin, sucralose, aspartame, dextrose, fructose and anything else you probably can't pronounce. Many of these can be very harsh on your gut and can still spike your blood sugar much like sugar does. Also, xylitol is highly toxic to dogs, so I don't recommend keeping this in your house if you have pets.

Stay Salty

Salt often gets a bad rap. But every chef knows how critical salt is to our food and how essential it is for our health too. And the best way to get all the salt and electrolytes you need is directly through your food. But not all salts are created equal, so here's some information to help you figure out the right salt for you, and when to use it.

Sea Salt and Pink Salt

Made from evaporated seawater, it is by far the most nutritious salt, due to its diverse mineral and electrolyte content. It has a complex flavor as well. I prefer Redmond Real Salt® made in the U.S., as it is free of microplastics, unlike many of the Himalayan salts mined abroad. But any sea salt or pink Himalayan salt is generally a great choice.

Kosher Salt

Due to its large crystal size, kosher salt is not as salty as table or sea salt by volume. If a recipe calls for sea salt, you can use kosher salt, but use about one-third extra to compensate for the lower salinity. It's also very inexpensive and is the preferred salt by restaurant chefs for its ease of use. It's also particularly good for seasoning a steak or fish, as the large crystals stick really nicely to raw meat.

Flaky Finishing Salt

Flaky salt is used on top of a finished dish, like steak. It's very expensive and has a large, pyramid-like structure. It adds not only flavor but texture to a dish and is only to be used at the end. There are flavor-infused finishing salts, as well. I love Maldon® Smoked Sea Salt for its wonderful smoky aroma.

Table Salt (Iodized)

This salt is very high in sodium—it's basically pure NaCl—low in nutritional value, and, frankly, it tastes terrible. Have you ever tasted it by itself? Yuck! Avoid using it in your cooking if you can, and leave it where it belongs: on the table, not in the kitchen.

Fat Is Your Friend

The various oils and fats each have unique smoke points—the temperature at which they start to burn. Using the right oil is important both for your cooking and for your health. Use the guide below to help you decide when and where to use various fats and oils.

Ingredient	Smoke Point	Suggested Use	Flavor
Butter	302°F (150°C)	Low heat, pan sauces, baking	Creamy, savory
Ghee	482°F (250°C)	Frying, searing, curries	Cheesy, bold
Vegetable, Canola, Peanut, Grapeseed Oils	400°F (204°C)–453°F (234°C)	Avoid using these, due to inflammatory properties	Neutral
Avocado Oil	520°F (271°C)	High-heat frying and deep frying	Mild, nutty
Olive Oil	320°F (160°C)	Roasting, using cold and in dressings	Fruity, spicy, flavorful
Animal Fat (Bacon, Lard, Tallow)	370–400°F (188–204°C)	Roasting, panfrying, deep frying	Flavorful, complex
Coconut Oil	350°F (177°C)	Sautéing, roasting, curries	Coconut flavor
Sesame Oil	350°F (177°C)	Finishing, best used raw and in dressings	Intense, nutty

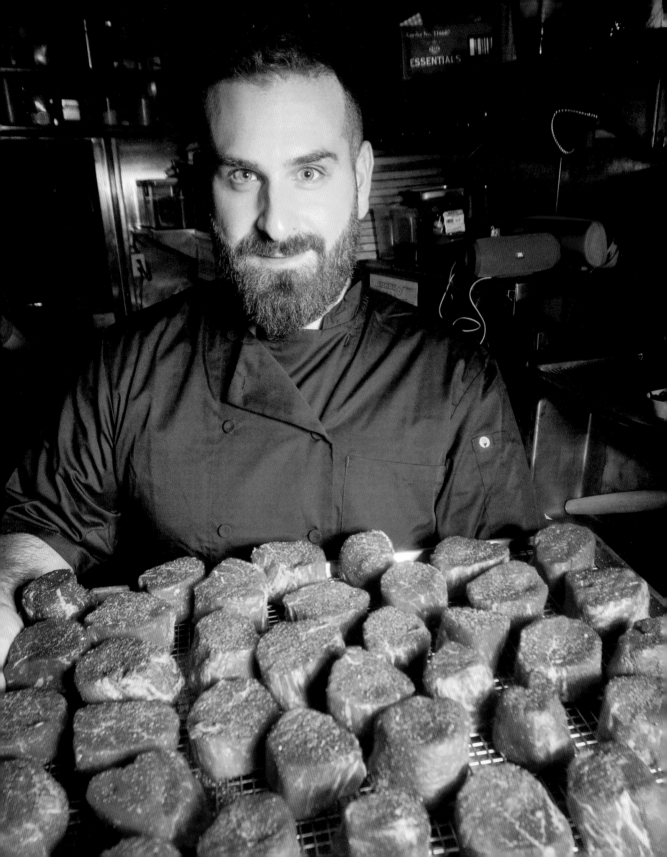

meat matters

I want you to get restaurant-quality results every time you cook. And you don't always need to buy the most expensive cut of meat to get amazing results. So here are a few tips for the juiciest, tenderest meat and seafood at home.

Relaxed and Ready

You may notice that throughout this book I've left instructions in the recipes for letting your meat "temper" before cooking. This simply means leaving it out on your countertop for 10 or 15 minutes before cooking. Pulling it out of the fridge ahead allows the meat to warm a bit before cooking. And this means the meat won't be so "shocked" when it hits the hot pan or oven. That temperature shock causes the meat fibers to tense up and will lead to tougher, dryer meat in the end.

Getting the Goods

The meat department can get overwhelming, so how do you know what to pick? Well, first of all, I would generally stay away from anything labeled "Select." "Choice" or, better-yet, "Prime" are great options. But that doesn't mean you need to break the bank on grass-fed, dry-aged, or Wagyu (the top-shelf of beef). Just remember: Choice or Prime, and you'll be fine. There are also some other ways of quickly identifying the best selection of a given steak just by looking at it. Look for meat that has noticeable marbling. The marbling will ensure a certain level of fat content inside the meat that will keep it nice and juicy as it cooks. Also consider how thick the steaks are. Really thick, and it'll be difficult getting it properly cooked; too thin and it'll get dry and tough very quickly. For chicken, fish and pork, look for meat that is firm, fresh and vibrant in color, and please avoid gray or slimy-looking chicken. And of course, get to know the folks at the meat counter. If you can't find a particular cut you're looking for, just ask!

Secrets of Seafood

I've generally found that larger shrimp just taste better and have a better texture—more like lobster—but jumbo shrimp can be very costly. Save money by buying frozen, easy-peel shrimp rather than the thawed and peeled shrimp at the seafood counter. Fun fact: Almost all shrimp at supermarkets in the U.S. are previously frozen, unless you live right next to the ocean. Quickly thaw frozen shrimp by letting them soak in a bowl of cool water for 15 minutes. If you're in a hurry and don't have time to peel your own shrimp (which is totally understandable!), just splurge for the ready-to-cook/peeled variety. And if you're looking for high-quality shrimp, look for locally sourced, or even better, wild-caught. However, when it comes to fish and other shellfish, there is simply no doubt that the fresher the better. Unlike shrimp, previously frozen fish can get really "fishy" tasting. So if there is one place I highly recommend spending a little extra, it's on fish. The only exception to this is sushi-grade fish, which you actually want to buy frozen.

Trash to Treasure

Don't let any of your bones, shrimp shells or vegetable trimmings go to waste! Whenever you're peeling shrimp, trimming meat or cutting veggies, save the scraps in zipper bags in the freezer. Once the bags are full, add them to a large soup pot, fill it with just enough water to cover the trimmings and boil for 1 to 2 hours. Season generously with sea salt, strain and sip on a nutrient-packed homemade bone broth.

Resting Is Required

If you haven't heard it a million times before, I'm going to tell you again: LET YOUR MEAT REST BEFORE SLICING IT. Okay, I'm sorry I yelled at you . . . but this is really important stuff. Resting your meat ensures that all the yummy juices stay inside the meat, rather than on your cutting board. A good rule of thumb is to let the meat rest for at least half as long as you cooked it. So if your steak took 10 minutes to cook, let it rest for a minimum of 5 minutes. Pinky swear you'll do this?

Meat Temperature Guide

Below are the recommended minimum internal temperatures for the various types of meat. The easiest way to guarantee perfectly cooked meat every time is to use a meat thermometer or instant-read thermometer. You can buy them inexpensively online if you don't have one. Just remember to take the internal temperature at the thickest, most central point in the meat for the most accurate reading.

Beef*	Steak (Flank, Strip, Ribeye, Porterhouse, T-bone)	130°F (54°C)
	Filet Mignon	125°F (52°C)
	Prime Rib	120°F (49°C)
	Meatloaf	160°F (71°C)
	Burgers	135°F (57°C)
Pork*	Pork Chops	140°F (60°C)
	Tenderloin	135°F (57°C)
Chicken	All Chicken	165°F (74°C)
Fish	Salmon	120°F (49°C)
	All Other Fish	140°F (60°C)
Game Meats*	Lamb and Goat	125°F (52°C)
	Duck Breast	130°F (54°C)
	Veal	135°F (57°C)
	Rabbit	145°F (63°C)
	Venison	135°F (57°C)

*Note: These temperatures are for medium-rare. For medium temperatures, add 5°F (15°C). According to the USDA, consuming raw or undercooked meats, poultry, seafood, shellfish or eggs may increase your risk of foodborne illness, especially if you are pregnant or have certain medical conditions.

knife life

We chefs live for our knives, but it can definitely seem pretty daunting to a home cook. And you really don't need a fancy, expensive knife set to be proficient in the kitchen. Here are a few tips for getting your chopping in order.

One and Done

All you need is one good-quality chef's knife to do pretty much everything in the kitchen. You can get a nice chef's knife for $50 to $100 USD, and it's worth every penny. Don't buy a huge knife set for hundreds of dollars. If you go to www.chef-michael.com/tools, you can find a short list of decent knives I recommend for anyone at any price point. And use a size you're comfortable and confident with. I think a 6- to 8-inch (15- to 20-cm) chef's knife or santoku-style knife is ideal.

Proper Protocols

First, use only a plastic or wooden cutting board—glass cutting boards will damage your knife's blade. Second, never run a good knife through the dishwasher, as it's the quickest way to dull and ruin your knife. And similarly, don't leave it at the bottom of your sink to get damaged or rusty. Set it aside on your countertop when you're done cooking, and quickly wash it after with soap and water. Then set it aside to air dry before storing. Just make sure they aren't loose in a drawer, which will bang up the edges. A knife block works great.

Staying Sharp

Ironically, a very sharp knife is the best way to prevent yourself from getting cut, as a dull knife can easily slip off the food you're slicing and land on a finger. So, keep your knife extra sharp. I send my knives out at least once a year to get professionally sharpened, and it usually costs about $10 per knife. Look for companies like KnifeAid online and you can just mail your knives out for sharpening right from home.

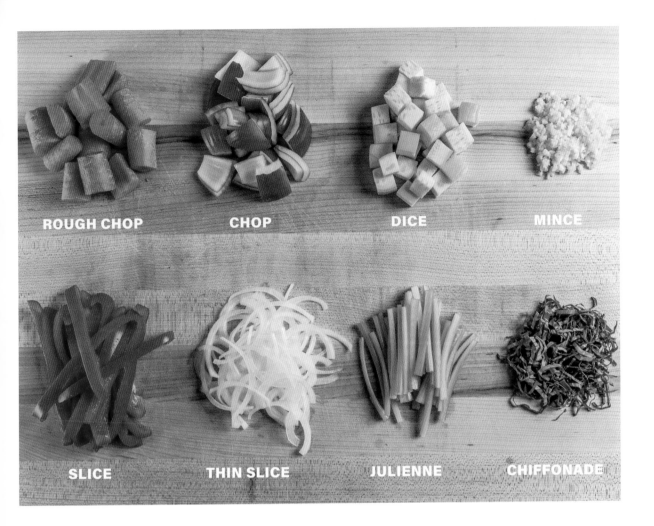

ROUGH CHOP CHOP DICE MINCE

SLICE THIN SLICE JULIENNE CHIFFONADE

Slice and Dice

Do you need to cut like Gordon Ramsay? No. But getting comfortable with a knife is a good idea. I'd suggest getting a cheap bag of onions or green peppers, and spend an hour practicing. You'll surprise yourself with how quickly you can become a master slicer and dicer. Use this diagram when you practice your knife skills to nail all the classic culinary cuts. You can also reference this photo anytime you're using my recipes, so when I call for something to be minced, diced or chopped, you'll know the difference.

acknowledgments

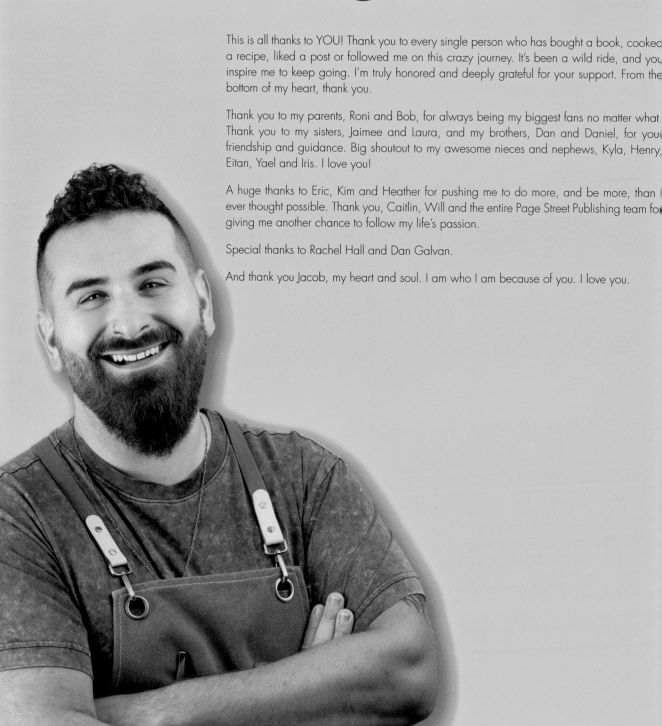

This is all thanks to YOU! Thank you to every single person who has bought a book, cooked a recipe, liked a post or followed me on this crazy journey. It's been a wild ride, and you inspire me to keep going. I'm truly honored and deeply grateful for your support. From the bottom of my heart, thank you.

Thank you to my parents, Roni and Bob, for always being my biggest fans no matter what. Thank you to my sisters, Jaimee and Laura, and my brothers, Dan and Daniel, for your friendship and guidance. Big shoutout to my awesome nieces and nephews, Kyla, Henry, Eitan, Yael and Iris. I love you!

A huge thanks to Eric, Kim and Heather for pushing me to do more, and be more, than I ever thought possible. Thank you, Caitlin, Will and the entire Page Street Publishing team for giving me another chance to follow my life's passion.

Special thanks to Rachel Hall and Dan Galvan.

And thank you Jacob, my heart and soul. I am who I am because of you. I love you.

about the author

As a bestselling author, blogger and TV personality, Michael Silverstein is passionate about the power of cooking to improve one's life. After losing more than 80 pounds (36 kg) in one year on the Ketogenic diet, Michael enthusiastically believes that health starts in the kitchen. And he hopes to continue helping others make incredible food at home while finding joy and empowerment through their cooking.

After beating out tens of thousands of competitors on Season 10 of *MasterChef*, he then returned to battle on the all-star Season 12 of *MasterChef*, proving once again that he is one of the best cooks in America.

Michael is the bestselling author of *New Keto Cooking* and *New Comfort Cooking*, and has been featured in *People*, *New York Post*, *National Examiner*, *Closer Weekly*, *Delish*, *Medium*, *FeedFeed* and *Diply*, and on the Hallmark Channel, *E! News* and more.

When he's not in the kitchen, Michael enjoys sipping on espresso, gardening, doing DIY projects, playing piano, traveling and exploring the Texas food scene. He lives in Austin with his fiancé, Jacob, their rescue dog, Meelo, and Duchess the cat.

For more of his recipes, find Michael on Instagram @chefmichael.keto, on TikTok @chef.michael or on his website chef-michael.com. And be sure to pick up a copy of his other books at any major retailer.

index

A

air fryer dishes
  Extra-Crispy Salmon and Green Beans with "Horsey" Sauce, 86
  My Big Fat Greek Sheet-Pan Chicken, 54
  The Perfect Garlic Parmesan Wings, 42
  Popcorn Pork Belly with Yum Yum Sauce, 62
allulose, 151
almond butter, in Chewy Ginger Almond Butter Cookies, 143
almond flour
  Blueberry Lemon Mini Muffins, 140
  Boozy Margarita Mug Cake, 136
  Firecracker Chicken Meatballs, 41
almonds, in Loaded Lemon-Pepper Broccoli Salad, 111
Amazing Keto Pork Fried Rice, 69
anchovy paste, in The Ultimate Blackened Chicken Caesar Salad, 107
andouille sausage, in Kickin' Cajun Shrimp and Sausage Bake, 85
arugula, in Steak and Avocado Salad with Sweet Onion Dressing, 108
asparagus
  Blue Cheese Lovers' Steak and Asparagus Sauté, 33
  Cheesy Baked Asparagus, 118
  Lemon Dill Salmon en Papillote, 93
Austin Food Truck Breakfast Tacos (for Dinner!), 65
avocado
  Steak and Avocado Salad with Sweet Onion Dressing, 108
  Summery Grilled Swordfish with Avocado Salsa, 81

B

bacon
  Austin Food Truck Breakfast Tacos (for Dinner!), 65
  Bacon Cheeseburger Skillet with "Big Mike" Sauce, 17
  Blissful Burrata and Pancetta Salad with Summer Citronette, 115
  Fabulous Bacon-Fried Cabbage Steaks, 133
  Loaded Lemon-Pepper Broccoli Salad, 111
  Low-Carb Barbecue Chicken Tortilla Pizzas, 49
Bacon Cheeseburger Skillet with "Big Mike" Sauce, 17
balsamic vinegar
  Beautifully Layered Eggplant Caprese, 129
  Blue Cheese Lovers' Steak and Asparagus Sauté, 33
  Sweet Balsamic-Glazed Brussels, 121
Banana Peppers, Spicy Italian Stuffed, 66
barbecue sauce, in Low-Carb Barbecue Chicken Tortilla Pizzas, 49
basil, Thai
  Thai Green Curry in a Hurry, 53
  Vibrant Thai-Style Pork Larb, 73
basil pesto, in Beautifully Layered Eggplant Caprese, 129
Beautifully Layered Eggplant Caprese, 129
beef
  about, 12; temperature guide for cooking, 155
  Bacon Cheeseburger Skillet with "Big Mike" Sauce, 17
  Blue Cheese Lovers' Steak and Asparagus Sauté, 33
  15-Minute Heavenly Steak Bites, 21
  Finger-Lickin' Low-Carb Steak Tacos with Smoky Crema, 26
  Hearty Stuffed Pepper Soup, 100
  Keto Korean Barbecue Short Ribs (L.A. galbi), 30
  Mediterranean-Spiced Kebabs with Dill Yogurt Drizzle, 34
  Mellow Mushroom Smothered Tri-Tips, 29
  Mouthwatering Mongolian Beef, 18
  No-Frilly Weeknight Chili, 22
  Steak and Avocado Salad with Sweet Onion Dressing, 108
  Texas Chili-Rubbed Ribeye with Fiery Chipotle Butter, 14
  Thousand Island Reuben Skillet, 25
beef broth
  Hearty Stuffed Pepper Soup, 100
  Mellow Mushroom Smothered Tri-Tips, 29
  No-Frilly Weeknight Chili, 22
bell peppers
  Austin Food Truck Breakfast Tacos (for Dinner!), 65
  Hearty Stuffed Pepper Soup, 100
  Kickin' Cajun Shrimp and Sausage Bake, 85
  Mediterranean-Spiced Kebabs with Dill Yogurt Drizzle, 34
  Thai Green Curry in a Hurry, 53
"Big Mike" Sauce, 17
blackening seasoning
  about: making own, 107
  The Ultimate Blackened Chicken Caesar Salad, 107
Blissful Burrata and Pancetta Salad with Summer Citronette, 115
Blistered Sichuan-Style Green Beans, 122
Blue Cheese Lovers' Steak and Asparagus Sauté, 33
Blueberry Lemon Mini Muffins, 140
Boozy Margarita Mug Cake, 136
bourbon, in Mike's Famous Bourbon Chicken, 38
broccoli
  Amazing Keto Pork Fried Rice, 69
  Lemony Spice-Roasted Mixed Veggies, 130
  Loaded Lemon-Pepper Broccoli Salad, 111
  Thai Green Curry in a Hurry, 53

russels Sprouts, Sweet Balsamic-Glazed, 121

urrata cheese, in Blissful Burrata and Pancetta Salad with Summer Citronette, 115

C

abbage, in Fabulous Bacon-Fried Cabbage Steaks, 133

ajun seasoning
    Kickin' Cajun Shrimp and Sausage Bake, 85
    Pork Chops in Wicked Mardi Gras Sauce, 74

anned and dry goods, list of basic, 150

apers, in Parmesan-Crusted Chicken Piccata, 57

auliflower (riced), in Fab 5-Minute Spanish Rice, 125

heddar cheese
    Austin Food Truck Breakfast Tacos (for Dinner!), 65
    Bacon Cheeseburger Skillet with "Big Mike" Sauce, 17
    Loaded Lemon-Pepper Broccoli Salad, 111
    Low-Carb Barbecue Chicken Tortilla Pizzas, 49

heesy Baked Asparagus, 118

hewy Ginger Almond Butter Cookies, 143

hicken
    about, 36; temperature guide for cooking, 155
    Chili-Lime Grilled Chicken with Garlicky Aioli, 58
    Firecracker Chicken Meatballs, 41
    Low-Carb Barbecue Chicken Tortilla Pizzas, 49
    Mike's Famous Bourbon Chicken, 38
    My Big Fat Greek Sheet-Pan Chicken, 54
    Parmesan-Crusted Chicken Piccata, 57
    The Perfect Garlic Parmesan Wings, 42
    Piece-of-Cake Chicken Bake, 45

Quick Chicken Parm, 50
Thai Green Curry in a Hurry, 53
The Ultimate Blackened Chicken Caesar Salad, 107
Vibrant Thai-Style Pork Larb, 73
Zesty "Honey Mustard" Chicken, 46

chicken bouillon powder
    Easy Egg Drop Soup, 99
    Fab 5-Minute Spanish Rice, 125
    Parmesan-Crusted Chicken Piccata, 57
    Simply Delish Sausage and Kale Soup, 104

Chili-Lime Grilled Chicken with Garlicky Aioli, 58

Chili, No-Frilly Weeknight, 22

Chili-Rubbed Ribeye with Fiery Chipotle Butter, 14

Chipotle Butter, 14

chipotle peppers in adobo sauce
    Finger-Lickin' Low-Carb Steak Tacos with Smoky Crema, 26
    Texas Chili-Rubbed Ribeye with Fiery Chipotle Butter, 14

chipotle powder, in Chili-Lime Grilled Chicken with Garlicky Aioli, 58

chocolate chips (sugar-free), in Mike's Midnight Munchie Bars, 144

cilantro
    about: using stems of, 58
    Chili-Lime Grilled Chicken with Garlicky Aioli, 58
    Summery Grilled Swordfish with Avocado Salsa, 81
    Texas Chili-Rubbed Ribeye with Fiery Chipotle Butter, 14
    Vibrant Thai-Style Pork Larb, 73

coconut cream
    Pork Chops in Wicked Mardi Gras Sauce, 74
    Zesty "Honey Mustard" Chicken, 46

coconut flakes, in Mike's Midnight Munchie Bars, 144

coconut flour, in Blueberry Lemon Mini Muffins, 140

coconut milk, in Thai Green Curry in a Hurry, 53

Colby cheese, in Low-Carb Barbecue Chicken Tortilla Pizzas, 49

Comforting Keto Cream of Mushroom Soup, 103

condiments and oils, list of basic, 150

Cookies, Chewy Ginger Almond Butter, 143

corned beef, in Thousand Island Reuben Skillet, 25

cream cheese
    Comforting Keto Cream of Mushroom Soup, 103
    Spinach and Artichoke Dip, 45

Creamy Sun-Dried Tomato Tuscan Shrimp, 78

cucumbers, in Date Night Spicy Tuna Sushi Boats, 82

D

Date Night Spicy Tuna Sushi Boats, 82

dill
    Lemon Dill Salmon en Papillote, 93
    Mediterranean-Spiced Kebabs with Dill Yogurt Drizzle, 34
    Protein-Packed Maryland Shrimp Salad, 112

dressings
    Caesar, 107
    Summer Citronette, 115
    Sweet Onion, 108
    Thousand Island, 25
    see also sauces

E

Easy Egg Drop Soup, 99

edamame spaghetti, in Luxurious Low-Carb Tuna Pasta with Olive Oil and Lemon, 89

Eggplant Caprese, Beautifully Layered, 129

eggs
    Amazing Keto Pork Fried Rice, 69
    Austin Food Truck Breakfast Tacos (for Dinner!), 65
    Blueberry Lemon Mini Muffins, 140

Chewy Ginger Almond Butter Cookies, 143

Easy Egg Drop Soup, 99

erythritol, 151

Extra-Crispy Salmon and Green Beans with "Horsey" Sauce, 86

F

Fab 5-Minute Spanish Rice, 125

Fabulous Bacon-Fried Cabbage Steaks, 133

fat, kinds of, described, 153

Feta cheese, in My Big Fat Greek Sheet-Pan Chicken, 54

15-Minute Heavenly Steak Bites, 21

Finger-Lickin' Low-Carb Steak Tacos with Smoky Crema, 26

Firecracker Chicken Meatballs, 41

fish, temperature guide for cooking, 155. *See also* seafood

fish sauce

Thai Green Curry in a Hurry, 53

Vibrant Thai-Style Pork Larb, 73

flaky finishing salt, 152

"Fool," Seductive Strawberry Mojito, 139

Frank's RedHot sauce, in Firecracker Chicken Meatballs, 41

G

game meats, temperature guide for, 155

garlic

Amazing Keto Pork Fried Rice, 69

Austin Food Truck Breakfast Tacos (for Dinner!), 65

Blistered Sichuan-Style Green Beans, 122

Blue Cheese Lovers' Steak and Asparagus Sauté, 33

Cheesy Baked Asparagus, 118

Comforting Keto Cream of Mushroom Soup, 103

Creamy Sun-Dried Tomato Tuscan Shrimp, 78

15-Minute Heavenly Steak Bites, 21

Hearty Stuffed Pepper Soup, 100

Keto Korean Barbecue Short Ribs (L.A. *galbi*), 30

Lemon Dill Salmon en Papillote, 93

Mellow Mushroom Smothered Tri-Tips, 29

Mouthwatering Mongolian Beef, 18

Parmesan-Crusted Chicken Piccata, 57

The Perfect Garlic Parmesan Wings, 42

Pork Chops in Wicked Mardi Gras Sauce, 74

Simply Delish Sausage and Kale Soup, 104

Succulent Spanish Garlic Shrimp (Gambas al Ajillo), 90

Texas Chili-Rubbed Ribeye with Fiery Chipotle Butter, 14

The Ultimate Blackened Chicken Caesar Salad, 107

Vibrant Thai-Style Pork Larb, 73

ginger

Amazing Keto Pork Fried Rice, 69

Blistered Sichuan-Style Green Beans, 122

Keto Korean Barbecue Short Ribs (L.A. *galbi*), 30

Mike's Famous Bourbon Chicken, 38

Mouthwatering Mongolian Beef, 18

Glaze, Tequila-Lime, 136

goat cheese, in Fabulous Bacon-Fried Cabbage Steaks, 133

Greek yogurt, in Mediterranean-Spiced Kebabs with Dill Yogurt Drizzle, 34

green beans

Blistered Sichuan-Style Green Beans, 122

Extra-Crispy Salmon and Green Beans with "Horsey" Sauce, 86

green curry paste, in Thai Green Curry in a Hurry, 53

H

Hearty Stuffed Pepper Soup, 100

heavy cream

Cheesy Baked Asparagus, 118

Comforting Keto Cream of Mushroom Soup, 103

Creamy Sun-Dried Tomato Tuscan Shrimp, 78

Mellow Mushroom Smothered Tri-Tips, 29

Pork Chops in Wicked Mardi Gras Sauce, 74

Seductive Strawberry Mojito Fool, 139

Zesty "Honey Mustard" Chicken, 46

Herby Pan-Roasted Mushrooms, 126

horseradish, in Extra-Crispy Salmon and Green Beans with "Horsey" Sauce, 86

Hungarian wax peppers, in Italian Stuffed Banana Peppers, 66

I

iodized table salt, 152

Irish-style butter

15-Minute Heavenly Steak Bites, 21

Luxurious Low-Carb Tuna Pasta with Olive Oil and Lemon, 89

Texas Chili-Rubbed Ribeye with Fiery Chipotle Butter, 14

Italian cheese blend

Cheesy Baked Asparagus, 118

Creamy Sun-Dried Tomato Tuscan Shrimp, 78

Italian parsley

Parmesan-Crusted Chicken Piccata, 57

The Perfect Garlic Parmesan Wings, 42

Succulent Spanish Garlic Shrimp (Gambas al Ajillo), 90

Italian sausage

Simply Delish Sausage and Kale Soup, 104

Spicy Italian Stuffed Banana Peppers, 66

J

jalapeños

Austin Food Truck Breakfast Tacos (for Dinner!), 65

No-Frilly Weeknight Chili, 22

Southwest Roasted Tomato Bisque, 96

Summery Grilled Swordfish with Avocado Salsa, 81

ale

about: using leftover, 104

Simply Delish Sausage and Kale Soup, 104

ebabs, Mediterranean-Spiced, with Dill Yogurt Drizzle, 34

eto Korean Barbecue Short Ribs (L.A. galbi), 30

ckin' Cajun Shrimp and Sausage Bake, 85

ives, care and use of, 156–157

osher salt, 152

rb, Vibrant Thai-Style, 73

st-Minute Low-Carb "Al Pastor" Bowls, 70

mon-Pepper Broccoli Salad, Loaded, 111

mons and lemon juice

Blissful Burrata and Pancetta Salad with Summer Citronette, 115

Blueberry Lemon Mini Muffins, 140

Fabulous Bacon-Fried Cabbage Steaks, 133

Kickin' Cajun Shrimp and Sausage Bake, 85

Lemon Dill Salmon en Papillote, 93

Lemony Spice-Roasted Mixed Veggies, 130

Luxurious Low-Carb Tuna Pasta with Olive Oil and Lemon, 89

Mediterranean-Spiced Kebabs with Dill Yogurt Drizzle, 34

My Big Fat Greek Sheet-Pan Chicken, 54

Parmesan-Crusted Chicken Piccata, 57

Succulent Spanish Garlic Shrimp (Gambas al Ajillo), 90

Thousand Island Reuben Skillet, 25

The Ultimate Blackened Chicken Caesar Salad, 107

lettuce

The Ultimate Blackened Chicken Caesar Salad, 107

Vibrant Thai-Style Pork Larb, 73

limes and lime juice

Boozy Margarita Mug Cake, 136

Chili-Lime Grilled Chicken with Garlicky Aioli, 58

Finger-Lickin' Low-Carb Steak Tacos with Smoky Crema, 26

Seductive Strawberry Mojito Fool, 139

Thai Green Curry in a Hurry, 53

Vibrant Thai-Style Pork Larb, 73

Loaded Lemon-Pepper Broccoli Salad, 111

Louisiana-Style hot sauce, in Pork Chops in Wicked Mardi Gras Sauce, 74

Low-Carb Barbecue Chicken Tortilla Pizzas, 49

Luxurious Low-Carb Tuna Pasta with Olive Oil and Lemon, 89

M

macadamia nuts, in Mike's Midnight Munchie Bars, 144

marinara sauce

Quick Chicken Parm, 50

Spicy Italian Stuffed Banana Peppers, 66

mayonnaise

Bacon Cheeseburger Skillet with "Big Mike" Sauce, 17

Chili-Lime Grilled Chicken with Garlicky Aioli, 58

Date Night Spicy Tuna Sushi Boats, 82

Extra-Crispy Salmon and Green Beans with "Horsey" Sauce, 86

Loaded Lemon-Pepper Broccoli Salad, 111

Popcorn Pork Belly with Yum Yum Sauce, 62

Protein-Packed Maryland Shrimp Salad, 112

The Ultimate Blackened Chicken Caesar Salad, 107

Meatballs, Firecracker Chicken, 41

meats

grades of, 154

resting before slicing, 155

temperature guide for cooking, 155

tempering of, 154

see also beef; chicken; pork

Mediterranean-Spiced Kebabs with Dill Yogurt Drizzle, 34

Mellow Mushroom Smothered Tri-Tips, 29

Mike's Famous Bourbon Chicken, 38

Mike's Midnight Munchie Bars, 144

mint leaves

Seductive Strawberry Mojito Fool, 139

Vibrant Thai-Style Pork Larb, 73

mise en place, 148

monk fruit, 151

Monterey Jack cheese, in Low-Carb Barbecue Chicken Tortilla Pizzas, 49

Mouthwatering Mongolian Beef, 18

mozzarella cheese

Beautifully Layered Eggplant Caprese, 129

Blissful Burrata and Pancetta Salad with Summer Citronette, 115

Cheesy Baked Asparagus, 118

Creamy Sun-Dried Tomato Tuscan Shrimp, 78

Piece-of-Cake Chicken Bake, 45

Quick Chicken Parm, 50

Spicy Italian Stuffed Banana Peppers, 66

muffins, Blueberry Lemon Mini Muffins, 140

Mug Cake, Boozy Margarita, 136

mushrooms

Comforting Keto Cream of Mushroom Soup, 103

Herby Pan-Roasted Mushrooms, 126

Lemony Spice-Roasted Mixed Veggies, 130

Mellow Mushroom Smothered Tri-Tips, 29

Simply Delish Sausage and Kale Soup, 104

Thai Green Curry in a Hurry, 53

mustard

Blissful Burrata and Pancetta Salad with Summer Citronette, 115

Extra-Crispy Salmon and Green Beans with "Horsey" Sauce, 86

Pork Chops in Wicked Mardi Gras Sauce, 74

Protein-Packed Maryland Shrimp Salad, 112

Steak and Avocado Salad with Sweet Onion Dressing, 108

The Ultimate Blackened Chicken Caesar Salad, 107

Zesty "Honey Mustard" Chicken, 46

My Big Fat Greek Sheet-Pan Chicken, 54

N

No-Frilly Weeknight Chili, 22

O

Old Bay seasoning

Kickin' Cajun Shrimp and Sausage Bake, 85

Protein-Packed Maryland Shrimp Salad, 112

olives, in My Big Fat Greek Sheet-Pan Chicken, 54

onions

Amazing Keto Pork Fried Rice, 69

Austin Food Truck Breakfast Tacos (for Dinner!), 65

Bacon Cheeseburger Skillet with "Big Mike" Sauce, 17

Comforting Keto Cream of Mushroom Soup, 103

Hearty Stuffed Pepper Soup, 100

Keto Korean Barbecue Short Ribs (L.A. *galbi*), 30

Kickin' Cajun Shrimp and Sausage Bake, 85

Low-Carb Barbecue Chicken Tortilla Pizzas, 49

Luxurious Low-Carb Tuna Pasta with Olive Oil and Lemon, 89

Mediterranean-Spiced Kebabs with Dill Yogurt Drizzle, 34

Mellow Mushroom Smothered Tri-Tips, 29

My Big Fat Greek Sheet-Pan Chicken, 54

No-Frilly Weeknight Chili, 22

Quick-Pickled Red Onions, 70

Simply Delish Sausage and Kale Soup, 104

Southwest Roasted Tomato Bisque, 96

Steak and Avocado Salad with Sweet Onion Dressing, 108

Summery Grilled Swordfish with Avocado Salsa, 81

Vibrant Thai-Style Pork Larb, 73

oranges and orange juice, in Blissful Burrata and Pancetta Salad with Summer Citronette, 115

P

pancetta, in Blissful Burrata and Pancetta Salad with Summer Citronette, 115

pantry, list of basic needs for, 150

Parmesan cheese

Cheesy Baked Asparagus, 118

Creamy Sun-Dried Tomato Tuscan Shrimp, 78

15-Minute Heavenly Steak Bites, 21

Luxurious Low-Carb Tuna Pasta with Olive Oil and Lemon, 89

Parmesan-Crusted Chicken Piccata, 57

The Perfect Garlic Parmesan Wings, 42

Piece-of-Cake Chicken Bake, 45

Quick Chicken Parm, 50

The Ultimate Blackened Chicken Caesar Salad, 107

pasta, Low-Carb Tuna Pasta with Olive Oil and Lemon, 89

pastrami, in Thousand Island Reuben Skillet, 25

pecans, in Blissful Burrata and Pancetta Salad with Summer Citronette, 115

pepper jack cheese, in Austin Food Truck Breakfast Tacos (for Dinner!), 65

pepperoncini, in My Big Fat Greek Sheet-Pan Chicken, 54

The Perfect Garlic Parmesan Wings, 42

Piece-of-Cake Chicken Bake, 45

pink salt, 152

Pizza, Low-Carb Barbecue Chicken Tortilla, 49

Popcorn Pork Belly with Yum Yum Sauce, 62

pork

about, 60; brining of, 74; temperature guide for, 155

Amazing Keto Pork Fried Rice, 69

Austin Food Truck Breakfast Tacos (for Dinner!), 65

Last-Minute Low-Carb "Al Pastor" Bowls, 70

Popcorn Pork Belly with Yum Yum Sauce, 62

Pork Chops in Wicked Mardi Gras Sauce, 74

Spicy Italian Stuffed Banana Pepper, 66

Vibrant Thai-Style Pork Larb, 73

Protein-Packed Maryland Shrimp Salad, 112

Q

Quick Chicken Parm, 50

R

red pepper flakes

Creamy Sun-Dried Tomato Tuscan Shrimp, 78

Firecracker Chicken Meatballs, 41

Low-Carb Barbecue Chicken Tortilla Pizzas, 49

The Perfect Garlic Parmesan Wings, 42

Piece-of-Cake Chicken Bake, 45

Simply Delish Sausage and Kale Soup, 104

Spicy Italian Stuffed Banana Peppers, 66

Succulent Spanish Garlic Shrimp (Gambas al Ajillo), 90

Vibrant Thai-Style Pork Larb, 73

en Skillet, Thousand Island, 25

in Amazing Keto Pork Fried Rice, . *See also* cauliflower (riced)

ed red peppers, in Southwest asted Tomato Bisque, 96

ds
about, 94
Blissful Burrata and Pancetta Salad with Summer Citronette, 115
Loaded Lemon-Pepper Broccoli Salad, 111
Protein-Packed Maryland Shrimp Salad, 112
Steak and Avocado Salad with Sweet Onion Dressing, 108
The Ultimate Blackened Chicken Caesar Salad, 107

on
Extra-Crispy Salmon and Green Beans with "Horsey" Sauce, 86
Lemon Dill Salmon en Papillote, 93

a, Avocado, 81

kinds of, 152

es
"Big Mike," 17
Firecreacker, 41
Garlic Parmesan, 42
Garlicky Cilantro Lime Aioli, 58
"Horsey," 86
Mardi Gras, 74
Smoky Chipotle Crema, 26
Yum Yum, 62
see also dressings

erkraut, in Thousand Island Reuben illet, 25

age
Kickin' Cajun Shrimp and Sausage Bake, 85
Simply Delish Sausage and Kale Soup, 104
Spicy Italian Stuffed Banana Peppers, 66

scallions
Amazing Keto Pork Fried Rice, 69
Date Night Spicy Tuna Sushi Boats, 82
Keto Korean Barbecue Short Ribs (L.A. *galbi*), 30
Loaded Lemon-Pepper Broccoli Salad, 111
Mouthwatering Mongolian Beef, 18
Vibrant Thai-Style Pork Larb, 73

sea salt, 152

seafood
about, 76, 154; thawing of frozen, 78, 82, 85, 90, 112, 154
Creamy Sun-Dried Tomato Tuscan Shrimp, 78
Date Night Spicy Tuna Sushi Boats, 82
Extra-Crispy Salmon and Green Beans with "Horsey" Sauce, 86
Kickin' Cajun Shrimp and Sausage Bake, 85
Lemon Dill Salmon en Papillote, 93
Luxurious Low-Carb Tuna Pasta with Olive Oil and Lemon, 89
Succulent Spanish Garlic Shrimp (Gambas al Ajillo), 90
Summery Grilled Swordfish with Avocado Salsa, 81

Seductive Strawberry Mojito Fool, 139

shallots
Succulent Spanish Garlic Shrimp (Gambas al Ajillo), 90
Vibrant Thai-Style Pork Larb, 73

sheet-pans, My Big Fat Greek Sheet-Pan Chicken, 54

shrimp
about: thawing of frozen, 78, 82, 85, 90, 112, 154
Creamy Sun-Dried Tomato Tuscan Shrimp, 78
Kickin' Cajun Shrimp and Sausage Bake, 85
Protein-Packed Maryland Shrimp Salad, 112
Succulent Spanish Garlic Shrimp (Gambas al Ajillo), 90

side dishes
about, 116
Beautifully Layered Eggplant Caprese, 129
Blistered Sichuan-Style Green Beans, 122
Cheesy Baked Asparagus, 118
Fab 5-Minute Spanish Rice, 125
Fabulous Bacon-Fried Cabbage Steaks, 133
Herby Pan-Roasted Mushrooms, 126
Lemony Spice-Roasted Mixed Veggies, 130
Sweet Balsamic-Glazed Brussels, 121

Simply Delish Sausage and Kale Soup, 104

soups
about, 94
Comforting Keto Cream of Mushroom Soup, 103
Easy Egg Drop Soup, 99
Hearty Stuffed Pepper Soup, 100
Simply Delish Sausage and Kale Soup, 104
Southwest Roasted Tomato Bisque, 96

sour cream
Blueberry Lemon Mini Muffins, 140
Finger-Lickin' Low-Carb Steak Tacos with Smoky Crema, 26

Southwest Roasted Tomato Bisque, 96

soy sauce
Amazing Keto Pork Fried Rice, 69
Blistered Sichuan-Style Green Beans, 122
Easy Egg Drop Soup, 99
Keto Korean Barbecue Short Ribs (L.A. *galbi*), 30
Mike's Famous Bourbon Chicken, 38
Mouthwatering Mongolian Beef, 18
Popcorn Pork Belly with Yum Yum Sauce, 62

spices and seasonings, list of basic, 150

spicy chili crisp
about, 69, 122

Blistered Sichuan-Style Green Beans, 122

Last-Minute Low-Carb "Al Pastor" Bowls, 69

Spicy Italian Stuffed Banana Peppers, 66

spinach

Blissful Burrata and Pancetta Salad with Summer Citronette, 115

Creamy Sun-Dried Tomato Tuscan Shrimp, 78

Piece-of-Cake Chicken Bake, 45

Spinach and Artichoke Dip, 45

squash, summer, in Lemony Spice-Roasted Mixed Veggies, 130

sriracha sauce

Date Night Spicy Tuna Sushi Boats, 82

Popcorn Pork Belly with Yum Yum Sauce, 62

Steak and Avocado Salad with Sweet Onion Dressing, 108

steak seasoning, in Blue Cheese Lovers' Steak and Asparagus Sauté, 33

stevia, 151

strawberries

Blissful Burrata and Pancetta Salad with Summer Citronette, 115

Seductive Strawberry Mojito Fool, 139

Succulent Spanish Garlic Shrimp (Gambas al Ajillo), 90

Summery Grilled Swordfish with Avocado Salsa, 81

Sweet Balsamic-Glazed Brussels, 121

sweeteners

alternatives to sugar, 151

best avoided, 151

sweets

about, 134

Blueberry Lemon Mini Muffins, 140

Boozy Margarita Mug Cake, 136

Chewy Ginger Almond Butter Cookies, 143

Mike's Midnight Munchie Bars, 144

Seductive Strawberry Mojito Fool, 139

Swiss cheese, in Thousand Island Reuben Skillet, 25

Swordfish, Summery Grilled, with Avocado Salsa, 81

T

table salt, 152

tacos

Austin Food Truck Breakfast Tacos (for Dinner!), 65

Finger-Lickin' Low-Carb Steak Tacos with Smoky Crema, 26

Texas Chili-Rubbed Ribeye with Fiery Chipotle Butter, 14

Thai Green Curry in a Hurry, 53

Thousand Island Reuben Skillet, 25

tips, tricks, and cooking basics

knives, 156

meats and, 154

pantry basics lists, 150

salts and, 152

to save money, 149–150

to save time, 148

sweeteners, 151

tomato paste

Hearty Stuffed Pepper Soup, 100

No-Frilly Weeknight Chili, 22

Popcorn Pork Belly with Yum Yum Sauce, 62

Pork Chops in Wicked Mardi Gras Sauce, 74

tomato sauce, in Fab 5-Minute Spanish Rice, 125

tomatoes, beefsteak

about: cutting of, 129

Beautifully Layered Eggplant Caprese, 129

tomatoes, fire-roasted diced

Hearty Stuffed Pepper Soup, 100

No-Frilly Weeknight Chili, 22

tomatoes, fresh

Kickin' Cajun Shrimp and Sausage Bake, 85

Lemony Spice-Roasted Mixed Veggies, 130

My Big Fat Greek Sheet-Pan Chicken, 54

Southwest Roasted Tomato Bisque, 96

Steak and Avocado Salad with Sweet Onion Dressing, 108

Summery Grilled Swordfish with Avocado Salsa, 81

tomatoes, sun-dried, in Creamy Tomato Tuscan Shrimp, 78

tortillas

Austin Food Truck Breakfast Tacos Dinner!), 65

Finger-Lickin' Low-Carb Steak Tacos with Smoky Crema, 26

Low-Carb Barbecue Chicken Tortilla Pizzas, 49

tuna

Date Night Spicy Tuna Sushi Boats, 82

Luxurious Low-Carb Tuna Pasta with Olive Oil and Lemon, 89

turkey, in Firecracker Meatballs, 41

U

The Ultimate Blackened Chicken Caesar Salad, 107

V

vegetable broth, in Comforting Keto Cream of Mushroom Soup, 103

Vibrant Thai-Style Pork Larb, 73

W

wine

Lemon Dill Salmon en Papillote, 9

Parmesan-Crusted Chicken Piccata, 57

wine vinegar, in Last-Minute Low-Carb Pastor" Bowls, 70

wings, The Perfect Garlic Parmesan Wings, 42

Worcestershire sauce, in Bacon Cheeseburger Skillet with "Big Mike Sauce, 17

Z

Zesty "Honey Mustard" Chicken, 46

zucchini, in Lemony Spice-Roasted Mixed Veggies, 130